PROCEDURE CHECKLISTS TO ACCOMPANY

Fundamentals of
NURSING

The Art and Science of Nursing Care

Fourth Edition

Carol Taylor, CSFN, RN, MSN, PhD
Director, Center for Clinical Bioethics
Assistant Professor, Nursing
Georgetown University
Washington, DC

Carol Lillis, RN, MSN
Interim Dean
Allied Health and Nursing
Delaware County Community College
Media, PA

Priscilla LeMone, RNC, DSN, FAAN
Associate Professor and Director
Undergraduate Program
Sinclair School of Nursing
University of Missouri–Columbia
Columbia, MO

Marilee LeBon, BA
Mountaintop, PA

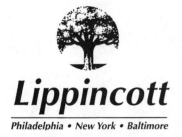

Lippincott

Philadelphia • New York • Baltimore

Ancillary Editor: Doris Wray
Senior Production Manager: Helen Ewan
Production Coordinator: Mike Carcel
Manufacturing Manager: William Alberti

Edition 4th

9 8 7 6 5 4 3 2 1

ISBN: 0-7817-2642-5

Care has been taken to confirm the accuracy of the information presented and to describe generally accepted practices. However, the authors, editors, and publisher are not responsible for errors or omissions or for any consequences from application of the information in this book and make no warranty, express or implied, with respect to the content of the publication.

The authors, editors, and publisher have exerted every effort to ensure that drug selection and dosage set forth in this text are in accordance with the current recommendations and practice at the time of publication. However, in view of ongoing research, changes in government regulations, and the constant flow of information relating to drug therapy and drug reactions, the reader is urged to check the package insert for each drug for any change in indications and dosage and for added warnings and precautions. This is particularly important when the recommended agent is a new or infrequently employed drug.

Some drugs and medical devices presented in this publication have Food and Drug Administration (FDA) clearance for limited use in restricted research settings. It is the responsibility of the health care provider to ascertain the FDA status of each drug or device planned for use in his or her clinical practice.

INTRODUCTION

Developing clinical competency is a major challenge for each fundamentals student. To facilitate the mastery of nursing procedures, we are happy to provide Procedure Checklists for each procedure in *Fundamentals of Nursing: The Art and Science of Nursing Care.* The Procedure Checklists follow each step of the procedure to provide a complete evaluative tool. Students can use the checklists to facilitate self-evaluation, and faculty will find them useful in measuring and recording student performance. Three-hole punched and perforated, these checklists can be easily reproduced and brought to the simulation laboratory or clinical area.

The checklists are designed to record an evaluation of each step of the procedure.

- Check mark in the "E" (excellent) column denotes mastering the procedure.
- Check mark in the "S" (satisfactory) column indicates use of the recommended technique.
- Check mark in the "NP" (needs practice) column indicates use of *some but not all* of each recommended technique.

The comments section allows you to highlight suggestions that will improve skills. Space is available at the bottom of each checklist to record a final pass/fail evaluation, date, and the signature of the student and evaluating faculty member.

LIST OF PROCEDURES

TABLE OF CONTENTS IN ALPHABETICAL ORDER

Procedure Checklists to Accompany Taylor Fundamentals of Nursing: The Art and Science of Nursing Care, 4th Edition

Name _____ Date _____

Unit _____ Position _____

Instructor/Evaluator _____ Position _____

Procedure 24-1

Assessing Body Temperature

Goal: To measure body heat for comparison with accepted normal values.

Excellent ▼	Satisfactory ▼	Needs Practice ▼		COMMENTS
___	___	___	1. Identify patient.	
___	___	___	2. Explain procedure to patient.	
___	___	___	3. Gather equipment.	
___	___	___	4. Wash your hands and don gloves if appropriate/indicated.	
___	___	___	5. Select appropriate site.	
___	___	___	6. Follow steps as outlined below for appropriate type of thermometer.	
___	___	___	7. Wash your hands. If wearing gloves, discard them in proper receptacle.	
___	___	___	8. Record temperature on paper, flow sheet, or computerized record. Report abnormal findings to the appropriate person. Identify assessment site if other than oral.	
			Assessing Tympanic Membrane Temperature	
___	___	___	1. If necessary, push the "On" button and wait for the "Ready" signal on unit.	
___	___	___	2. Attach tympanic probe cover.	
___	___	___	3. Using gentle but firm pressure, insert probe snugly into external ear.	
___	___	___	4. Activate unit by pushing trigger button. Reading is immediate, usually within 2 seconds.	
___	___	___	5. Note temperature reading. Discard probe cover and replace thermometer in its charger or holder.	

Excellent	Satisfactory	Needs Practice	
			## *Procedure 24-1*
			# Assessing Body Temperature (continued)
▼	▼	▼	**Goal:** To measure body heat for comparison with accepted normal values. **COMMENTS**
			Assessing Oral Temperature with Glass Thermometer
——	——	——	1. If stored in a chemical solution, wipe thermometer dry with a soft tissue, using a firm twisting motion. Wipe from bulb toward fingers.
——	——	——	2. Grasp thermometer firmly with the thumb and forefinger. Using strong wrist movements, shake it until the mercury line reaches at least 36° C (96.8° F).
——	——	——	3. Read thermometer by holding it horizontally at eye level and rotating it between the fingers until the mercury line is clearly visualized.
——	——	——	4. Place thermometer's mercury bulb within the back of the right or left pocket under patient's tongue. Tell patient to close lips around thermometer.
——	——	——	5. Leave thermometer in place for 3 minutes or according to agency protocol.
——	——	——	6. Remove thermometer. Using a firm, twisting motion, wipe it once from fingers down to mercury bulb.
——	——	——	7. Read thermometer to nearest tenth.
——	——	——	8. Dispose of tissues in a receptacle for contaminated items.
——	——	——	9. Wash thermometer in lukewarm soapy water. Rinse it in cool water. Dry and replace thermometer in its container.
			Assessing Rectal Temperature Using Glass Thermometer
——	——	——	1. Don gloves.
——	——	——	2. Wipe, shake, and read rectal thermometer.
——	——	——	3. Lubricate mercury bulb to about 2.5 cm (1 inch) up the stem.
——	——	——	4. Provide privacy. With patient lying on side and buttocks exposed, separate buttocks so anal sphincter is seen clearly.
——	——	——	5. Insert thermometer for approximately 3.8 cm (1-1/2 inches) in an adult, 2.5 cm (1 inch) in a child, and 1.25 cm (1/2 inch) in an infant.
——	——	——	6. Holding thermometer in place, let buttocks fall into place. Continue holding thermometer for 2–3 minutes.
——	——	——	7. Remove thermometer. Wipe it once with soft tissue from fingers to mercury bulb, using firm twisting motion.

Procedure 24-1

Assessing Body Temperature (continued)

Excellent ▼	Satisfactory ▼	Needs Practice ▼	**Goal:** To measure body heat for comparison with accepted normal values.	COMMENTS
___	___	___	8. Wipe anus of any feces and remaining lubricant.	
___	___	___	9. Read thermometer and dispose of tissue and gloves in proper receptacle. (Remove gloves from inside out.)	
___	___	___	10. Wash thermometer in lukewarm soapy water. Rinse in cool water. Dry and replace thermometer in a container labeled "rectal thermometer."	
			Assessing Axillary Temperature Using Glass Thermometer	
___	___	___	1. Move clothing to expose axilla.	
___	___	___	2. Place thermometer bulb in the center of axilla and bring patient's arm down close to the body.	
___	___	___	3. Remain with patient and leave thermometer in place for 10 minutes.	
			Assessing Temperature with Electronic Thermometer	
___	___	___	1. Release electronic unit from charging unit and remove probe from within recording unit.	
___	___	___	2. Cover thermometer probe with disposable probe cover and slide until it snaps into place.	
___	___	___	3. For rectal temperatures, lubricate probe.	
___	___	___	4. Place probe in posterior sublingual pocket and ask patient to close lips around probe (oral). Or insert in rectum as described when using a glass thermometer (rectal). Or place in center of axilla with arm against chest wall (axillary).	
___	___	___	5. Hold probe in place until an audible signal sounds.	
___	___	___	6. Note temperature reading and dispose of probe cover by pressing probe release button while holding probe over a receptacle.	
___	___	___	7. Replace thermometer in its charger/holder.	

Procedure Checklists to Accompany Taylor Fundamentals of Nursing: The Art and Science of Nursing Care, 4th Edition

Name _____ Date _____

Unit _____ Position _____

Instructor/Evaluator _____ Position _____

Excellent	Satisfactory	Needs Practice	Procedure 24-2 **Assessing Respiratory Rate**	COMMENTS
			Goal: To measure pulmonary ventilation for comparison with accepted normal values.	
——	——	——	1. While your fingers are still in place after counting the pulse rate, observe patient's respirations.	
——	——	——	2. Note rise and fall of patient's chest.	
——	——	——	3. Using watch with a second hand, count number of respirations for a minimum of 30 seconds. Multiply this number by 2 for respiratory rate per minute.	
——	——	——	4. If respirations are abnormal in any way, count respirations for at least 1 full minute.	
——	——	——	5. Document respiratory rate on paper, flow sheet, or computerized record. Report any abnormal findings to appropriate person.	
——	——	——	6. Wash your hands.	

Procedure Checklists to Accompany Taylor Fundamentals of Nursing: The Art and Science of Nursing Care, 4th Edition

Name _____ Date _____

Unit _____ Position _____

Instructor/Evaluator _____ Position _____

Procedure 24-3

Assessing Pulse

Goal: To measure heart rate for comparison with accepted normal values.

Excellent	Satisfactory	Needs Practice		COMMENTS
▼	▼	▼		
___	___	___	1. Identify patient.	
___	___	___	2. Explain procedure to patient.	
___	___	___	3. Gather equipment.	
___	___	___	4. Wash your hands and don gloves as appropriate.	
___	___	___	5. Select appropriate site.	
___	___	___	6. Follow steps as outlined below for appropriate pulse assessment.	
___	___	___	7. Wash your hands.	
___	___	___	8. Record pulse rate and site on paper, flow sheet, or computerized record. Report abnormal findings to appropriate person. Identify assessment site if other than apical.	

Assessing Radial Pulse

___	___	___	1. Patient may either be supine with arm alongside body, wrist extended and palms down; or sitting with forearm at a 90 degree angle to body resting on a support with wrist extended and palm downward.	
___	___	___	2. Place your first, second, and third fingers along patient's radial artery and press gently against the radius. Rest your thumb on back of patient's wrist.	
___	___	___	3. Apply only enough pressure to distinctly feel the artery.	
___	___	___	4. Using watch with a second hand, count number of pulsations felt for 30 seconds. Multiply this number by 2 to have rate for 1 minute. If pulse's rate, rhythm, or amplitude are abnormal in any way, palpate for 1 minute longer.	

Procedure 24-3

Assessing Pulse (continued)

Goal: To measure heart rate for comparison
with accepted normal values.

Excellent	Satisfactory	Needs Practice		COMMENTS
▼	▼	▼		

Assessing the Apical Pulse Rate

——	——	——	1. Use alcohol swab to clean stethoscope ear pieces and diaphragm.
——	——	——	2. Assist patient to sit in chair or sit up in bed then expose upper chest area.
——	——	——	3. Hold stethoscope diaphragm against palm of your hand for a few seconds.
——	——	——	4. Palpate 5th intercostal space and move to left midclavicular line. Place diaphragm over apex of heart.
——	——	——	5. Listen for heart sounds identified as a "lub-dub" sound.
——	——	——	6. Using watch with a second hand, count heartbeat for 1 minute.

Procedure Checklists to Accompany Taylor Fundamentals of Nursing: The Art and Science of Nursing Care, 4th Edition

Name _____ Date _____

Unit _____ Position _____

Instructor/Evaluator _____ Position _____

Procedure 24-4

Assessing Blood Pressure

Goal: To measure force of blood against arterial walls for comparison with accepted normal values.

Excellent	Satisfactory	Needs Practice		COMMENTS
▼	▼	▼		
___	___	___	1. Identify patient.	
___	___	___	2. Explain procedure to patient.	
___	___	___	3. Gather equipment.	
___	___	___	4. Wash your hands.	
___	___	___	5. Follow procedure as outlined below.	
___	___	___	6. Wash your hands. If wearing gloves, discard them in proper receptacle.	
___	___	___	7. Record on paper, flow sheet, or computerized record. Report abnormal findings to appropriate person. Identify assessment site if other than brachial.	

Assessing Blood Pressure

___	___	___	1. Delay obtaining blood pressure if patient is emotionally upset, in pain, or has just exercised, unless it is urgent to obtain blood pressure.	
___	___	___	2. Select appropriate arm for application of cuff (no intravenous infusion, breast or axilla surgery, cast, arteriovenous shunt, or injured or diseased limb on that side).	
___	___	___	3. Have patient assume a comfortable lying or sitting position with forearm supported at the level of the heart and with palm upward.	
___	___	___	4. Expose area of brachial artery by removing garments or moving sleeve, if it is not too tight, above area where cuff will be placed.	
___	___	___	5. Center bladder of cuff over brachial artery approximately midway on arm, so lower edge of cuff is about 2.5–5 cm (1–2 inches) above inner aspect of elbow. Tubing should extend from cuff edge nearer patient's elbow.	

Procedure 24-4

Assessing Blood Pressure (continued)

Goal: To measure force of blood against arterial walls for comparison with accepted normal values.

Excellent	Satisfactory	Needs Practice		COMMENTS
▼	▼	▼		
——	——	——	6. Wrap cuff smoothly and snugly around arm. Fasten it securely or tuck end of cuff well under preceding wrapping. Do not allow any clothing to interfere with proper placement of cuff.	
——	——	——	7. Check that mercury manometer is in a vertical position. Mercury must be within the zero area with gauge at eye level. If using an aneroid gauge, needle should be within the zero mark.	
——	——	——	8. Palpate pulse at brachial or radial artery by pressing gently with fingertips.	
——	——	——	9. Tighten screw valve on air pump.	
——	——	——	10. Inflate cuff while continuing to palpate artery. Note point on gauge where pulse disappears.	
——	——	——	11. Deflate cuff and wait 15 seconds.	
——	——	——	12. Assume a position no more than 3 feet away from gauge.	
——	——	——	13. Place stethoscope earpieces in ears. Direct eartips forward into the canal and not against ear itself.	
——	——	——	14. Place stethoscope bell or diaphragm firmly but with as little pressure as possible over brachial artery. Do not allow stethoscope to touch clothing or cuff.	
——	——	——	15. Pump the pressure 30 mm Hg above point at which systolic pressure was palpated and estimated. Open manometer valve and allow air to escape slowly (allowing gauge to drop 2–3 mm per heartbeat).	
——	——	——	16. Note point on gauge at which the first faint, but clear, sound appears and slowly and increases in intensity. Note this number as the systolic pressure.	
——	——	——	17. Read pressure to the closest even number.	
——	——	——	18. Do not reinflate cuff once air is being released to recheck the systolic pressure reading.	
——	——	——	19. Note the pressure at which the sound first becomes muffled. Also observe point at which sound completely disappears. These may occur separately or at the same point.	
——	——	——	20. Allow remaining air to escape quickly. Repeat any suspicious reading, but wait 30–60 seconds between readings to allow normal circulation to return to limb. Be sure to deflate cuff completely between attempts to check blood pressure.	
——	——	——	21. Remove cuff. Clean and store equipment.	

Procedure Checklists to Accompany Taylor Fundamentals of Nursing: The Art and Science of Nursing Care, 4ᵗʰ Edition

Name _____ Date _____

Unit _____ Position _____

Instructor/Evaluator _____ Position _____

Excellent	Satisfactory	Needs Practice	
▼	▼	▼	

Procedure 26-1

Applying Restraints

Goal: To promote safety by limiting movement.   **COMMENTS**

Excellent	Satisfactory	Needs Practice	
___	___	___	1. Determine need for restraints. Assess patient's physical condition, behavior, and mental status.
___	___	___	2. Confirm agency policy for application of restraints. Secure a physician's order.
___	___	___	3. Explain reason for use to patient and family. Clarify how care will be given and needs will be met, and that use of restraints is a temporary measure.
___	___	___	4. Wash your hands.
___	___	___	5. Apply restraints according to manufacturer's directions.
___	___	___	a. Choose the least restrictive type of device to allow greatest possible degree of mobility.
___	___	___	b. Pad bony prominences.
___	___	___	c. For restraint applied to extremity, ensure that two fingers can be inserted between the restraints and patient's wrist or ankle.
___	___	___	d. Maintain restrained extremity in normal anatomic position.
___	___	___	e. Use appropriate tie for all restraints.
___	___	___	f. Fasten restraint to the bed frame, *not the side rail.* Site should not be readily accessible to the patient.
___	___	___	6. Remove restraint at least every 2 hours or according to agency policy and patient need.
___	___	___	a. Check for signs of decreased circulation or impaired skin integrity.
___	___	___	b. Perform range-of-motion exercise before reapplying.
___	___	___	7. Reassure patient at regular intervals. Have call bell within easy reach.

Excellent	Satisfactory	Needs Practice	
			## Procedure 26-1
			# Applying Restraints (continued)

Goal: To promote safety by limiting movement.   **COMMENTS**

Excellent	Satisfactory	Needs Practice	
——	——	——	8. Assess for signs of sensory deprivation, such as increased sleeping, day-dreaming, anxiety, panic, and hallucinations.
——	——	——	9. Wash your hands.
——	——	——	10. Document reason for restraining patient, alternative measures attempted before applying the restraint, date and time of application, type of restraint, times when removed, and result and frequency of nursing assessment every 2 hours. Obtain a new order after 24 hours if restraints are still necessary.

Procedure Checklists to Accompany Taylor Fundamentals of Nursing: The Art and Science of Nursing Care, 4ᵗʰ Edition

Name _____ Date _____

Unit _____ Position _____

Instructor/Evaluator _____ Position _____

Procedure 27-1

Handwashing

Goal: To prevent and control spread of infection.

Excellent	Satisfactory	Needs Practice		COMMENTS
▼	▼	▼		
___	___	___	1. Stand in front of sink. Do not allow your uniform to touch sink during the washing procedure.	
___	___	___	2. Remove jewelry, if possible, and secure in a safe place or allow plain wedding band to remain in place.	
___	___	___	3. Turn on water and adjust force. Regulate temperature until water is warm.	
___	___	___	4. Wet hands and wrist area. Keep hands lower than elbows to allow water to flow toward fingertips.	
___	___	___	5. Use about 1 teaspoon liquid soap (3–5 mL) from dispenser or rinse bar of soap and lather thoroughly. Cover all areas of hands with soap product. Rinse soap bar again and return to soap dish.	
___	___	___	6. With firm rubbing and circular motions, wash palms and backs of hands, each finger, the areas between fingers, knuckles, wrists, and forearms. Wash at least 1 inch above area of contamination. If hands are not visibly soiled, wash to 1 inch above the wrists.	
___	___	___	7. Continue this friction motion for 10–15 seconds.	
___	___	___	8. Use fingernails of the other hand or a clean orangewood stick to clean under fingernails.	
___	___	___	9. Rinse thoroughly.	
___	___	___	10. Beginning with fingers and moving upward toward forearms, dry hands with a paper towel and discard it immediately. Use another clean towel to turn off faucet. Discard towel immediately without touching other clean hand.	
___	___	___	11. Use lotion on hands if desired.	

Procedure Checklists to Accompany Taylor Fundamentals of Nursing: The Art and Science of Nursing Care, 4th Edition

Name _____ Date _____

Unit _____ Position _____

Instructor/Evaluator _____ Position _____

Procedure 27-2

Preparing a Sterile Field

Goal: To ensure maintenance of surgical asepsis.

Excellent	Satisfactory	Needs Practice		COMMENTS
▼	▼	▼		
——	——	——	1. Explain procedure to patient.	
——	——	——	2. Gather equipment.	
——	——	——	3. Wash your hands.	
——	——	——	4. Check that sterile wrapped drape of package is dry and unopened. Also note expiration date.	
——	——	——	5. Select a work area that is waist level or higher.	
——	——	——	6. Open sterile wrapped drape or commercially prepared sterile package.	
——	——	——	a. For sterile wrapped drape, open outer covering. Remove sterile drape, lifting it carefully by its corners. Shake open, hold away from your body, and lay drape on selected work area.	
——	——	——	b. Place commercially prepared package in center of work area. Touching outer surface only, carefully reach around item and fold topmost flap of wrapper away from you. Open right and left flap before grasping nearest flap and opening toward you.	
——	——	——	7. Place additional sterile items on field as needed.	
——	——	——	8. Open agency-prepared item or commercially packaged item.	
——	——	——	a. Hold agency-wrapped item in one hand with top flap opening away from you. With other hand, unfold top flap and both sides. Keeping a secure hold on item, grasp corners of wrapper and pull back toward wrist, covering hand and wrist.	
——	——	——	b. If commercially packaged item has an unsealed corner, hold package in one hand and pull back on top cover with other hand. If edge is partially sealed, use both hands to carefully pull apart.	

Procedure 27-2

Preparing a Sterile Field (continued)

Excellent	Satisfactory	Needs Practice	

Goal: To ensure maintenance of surgical asepsis.

COMMENTS

___ ___ ___ 9. Drop sterile item onto sterile field from a 6-inch (15 cm) height or add item to field from the side. Be careful to avoid 1-inch border.

___ ___ ___ 10. Discard wrapper.

___ ___ ___ 11. Obtain appropriate solution and check expiration date.

___ ___ ___ 12. Open solution container according to directions and place cap on table with edges up.

___ ___ ___ 13. If bottle has been previously opened, "lip" it by pouring a small amount of solution into waste container.

___ ___ ___ 14. Hold bottle outside the edge of the sterile field with the label side uppermost. Prepare to pour from a height of 4–6 inches (10–15 cm). Bottle tip should never touch a sterile container or dressing.

___ ___ ___ 15. Pour required amount of solution steadily into sterile container positioned at side of sterile field. Avoid splashing any liquid.

___ ___ ___ 16. Touch only the outside of the lid when recapping.

Procedure Checklists to Accompany Taylor Fundamentals of Nursing: The Art and Science of Nursing Care, 4th Edition

Name _____   Date _____

Unit _____   Position _____

Instructor/Evaluator _____   Position _____

Procedure 27-3

Donning and Removing Sterile Gloves

Goal: To provide an additional barrier against spread of infection.

Excellent ▼	Satisfactory ▼	Needs Practice ▼		COMMENTS
			To Don Gloves:	
⎯	⎯	⎯	1. Wash and dry hands carefully.	
⎯	⎯	⎯	2. Place sterile glove package on clean, dry surface above your waist.	
⎯	⎯	⎯	3. Open the outside wrapper by carefully peeling back top layer. Remove inner package, handling only the outside of it.	
⎯	⎯	⎯	4. Carefully open inner package and expose sterile gloves with the cuff closest to you.	
⎯	⎯	⎯	5. With thumb and forefinger of nondominant hand, grasp folded cuff of sterile glove for dominant hand.	
⎯	⎯	⎯	6. Lift and hold glove with fingers down. Be careful it does not touch any unsterile object.	
⎯	⎯	⎯	7. Carefully insert dominant hand into glove and pull glove on. Leave cuff folded down until other hand is gloved.	
⎯	⎯	⎯	8. Holding thumb outward, slide fingers of gloved hand under cuff of remaining glove and lift glove upward.	
⎯	⎯	⎯	9. Carefully insert nondominant hand into glove. Adjust gloves on both hands touching only sterile areas.	
			To Remove Gloves:	
⎯	⎯	⎯	1. Using dominant hand, grasp other glove near cuff end and remove by inverting it, keeping contaminated area on the inside. Continue to hold onto glove.	
⎯	⎯	⎯	2. Slide fingers of ungloved hand inside remaining glove. Grasp glove on inside and remove by turning inside out over hand and other glove.	
⎯	⎯	⎯	3. Discard gloves in appropriate container and wash hands.	

Procedure Checklists to Accompany Taylor Fundamentals of Nursing: The Art and Science of Nursing Care, 4ᵗʰ Edition

Name _____ Date _____

Unit _____ Position _____

Instructor/Evaluator _____ Position _____

Excellent	Satisfactory	Needs Practice		
▼	▼	▼	**Procedure 27-4** **Using Personal Protective Equipment** **Goal:** To minimize or prevent exposure to infectious material.	**COMMENTS**
___	___	___	1. Check physician's order for type of isolation and review precautions in Infection Control Manual.	
___	___	___	2. Plan nursing activities and gather necessary equipment prior to entering patient's room.	
___	___	___	3. Provide instruction about isolation precautions to patient, family members, and visitors.	
___	___	___	4. Wash your hands.	
___	___	___	5. Put on gown, gloves, mask and protective eyewear, if recommended, as isolation precaution.	
___	___	___	a. Tie gown securely at neck and waist.	
___	___	___	b. Use clean disposable gloves. If worn with a gown, draw glove cuffs over gown sleeves.	
___	___	___	c. Securely tie and fit mask to face.	
___	___	___	d. Wear eyewear with face shields or protection on side of face.	
___	___	___	6. When patient care is completed, remove gloves.	
___	___	___	a. Untie waist strings of gown. Grasp outside of one glove and turn inside out to remove. Continue to hold onto glove.	
___	___	___	b. Insert fingers of ungloved hand inside cuff of remaining glove. Grasp glove on inside and remove by turning inside out. Drop in appropriate container.	

Procedure 27-4

Using Personal Protective Equipment (continued)

Goal: To minimize or prevent exposure to infectious material.

Excellent	Satisfactory	Needs Practice		COMMENTS
▼	▼	▼		
―	―	―	7. After removing gloves, remove mask:	
			Surgical mask	
―	―	―	a. Untie mask and drop by strings into waste container.	
			Particulate mask	
―	―	―	b. Use hand to hold respirator in place.	
―	―	―	c. Pull bottom strap up and over head.	
―	―	―	d. Pull top strap over head.	
―	―	―	e. Remove respirator from face and save for future use or discard according to manufacturer's directions.	
―	―	―	8. Remove gown.	
―	―	―	a. Gown that is not visibly soiled requires no particular technique for removal.	
			For gown that is visibly soiled:	
―	―	―	b. Untie neck strings of gown. Remove gown without touching outside of gown by keeping one hand up and under gown cuff and using this protected hand to pull opposite sleeve down and off.	
―	―	―	c. Use ungowned arm and hand to grasp gown from the inside and remove from the remaining arm. Remove gown, turn inside out, and drop in appropriate container.	
―	―	―	9. Remove eyewear and clean according to agency policy.	
―	―	―	10. Wash hands thoroughly.	

Procedure Checklists to Accompany Taylor Fundamentals of Nursing: The Art and Science of Nursing Care, 4th Edition

Name _____ Date _____

Unit _____ Position _____

Instructor/Evaluator _____ Position _____

Excellent ▼	Satisfactory ▼	Needs Practice ▼	*Procedure 28-1* **Administering Oral Medications** **Goal:** To provide a safe, effective method of giving drugs intended for absorption in stomach and small intestine.	COMMENTS
___	___	___	1. Gather equipment. Check each medication order against original physician's order according to agency policy. Clarify any inconsistencies. Check patient's chart for allergies.	
___	___	___	2. Know actions, special nursing considerations, safe-dose ranges, purpose of administration, and adverse effects of medications to be administered.	
___	___	___	3. Wash your hands.	
___	___	___	4. Move medication cart outside patient's room or prepare for administration in medication area.	
___	___	___	5. Unlock medication cart or drawer.	
___	___	___	6. Prepare medications for one patient at a time.	
___	___	___	7. Select proper medication from drawer or stock and compare with Kardex or order. Check expiration dates and perform calculations if necessary.	
___	___	___	a. Place unit dose-packaged medications in a disposable cup. Do not open wrapper until at bedside. Keep narcotics and medications that require special nursing assessments in a separate container.	
___	___	___	b. When removing tablets or capsules from a bottle, pour the necessary number into bottle cap and then place tablets in a medication cup. Break only scored tablets, if necessary, to obtain proper dose.	
___	___	___	c. Hold liquid medication bottles with the label against palm. Use appropriate measuring device when pouring liquids and read the amount of medication at the bottom of the meniscus at eye level. Wipe bottle lip with a paper towel.	

Procedure 28-1

Administering Oral Medications (continued)

Goal: To provide a safe, effective method of giving drugs intended for absorption in stomach and small intestine.

Excellent ▼	Satisfactory ▼	Needs Practice ▼		COMMENTS
___	___	___	8. Recheck each medication package or preparation with the order as it is poured.	
___	___	___	9. When all medications for one patient have been prepared, recheck once again with the medication order before taking them to patient.	
___	___	___	10. Carefully transport medications to patient's bedside. Keep medications in sight at all times.	
___	___	___	11. See that patient receives medications at the correct time.	
___	___	___	12. Identify the patient carefully. There are three correct ways to do this:	
___	___	___	a. Check name on patient's identification bracelet.	
___	___	___	b. Ask patient his/her name.	
___	___	___	c. Verify patient's identification with a staff member who knows patient.	
___	___	___	13. Complete necessary assessments before administration of medications. Check allergy bracelet or ask patient about allergies. Explain purpose and action of each medication to patient.	
___	___	___	14. Assist patient to an upright or lateral position.	
___	___	___	15. Administer medications:	
___	___	___	a. Offer water or other permitted fluids with pills, capsules, tablets, and some liquid medications.	
___	___	___	b. Ask patient's preference regarding medications to be taken by hand or in a cup and one at a time or all at once.	
___	___	___	c. If capsule or tablet falls to the floor, discard it and administer a new one.	
___	___	___	d. Record any fluid intake if I-O measurement is ordered.	
___	___	___	16. Remain with patient until each medication is swallowed. Unless nurse has seen patient swallow drug, she cannot record drug as having been administered.	
___	___	___	17. Wash your hands.	

Procedure 28-1

Administering Oral Medications (continued)

Goal: To provide a safe, effective method of giving drugs intended for absorption in stomach and small intestine.

Excellent	Satisfactory	Needs Practice		COMMENTS
▼	▼	▼		
___	___	___	18. Record each medication given on medication chart or record using required format.	
___	___	___	a. If drug was refused or omitted, record this in appropriate area on medication record.	
___	___	___	b. Recording of administration of a narcotic requires additional documentation on a narcotic record stating drug count and other specific information.	
___	___	___	19. Check on patient within 30 minutes of drug administration to verify response to medication.	

Procedure Checklists to Accompany Taylor Fundamentals of Nursing: The Art and Science of Nursing Care, 4th Edition

Name _____ Date _____

Unit _____ Position _____

Instructor/Evaluator _____ Position _____

Procedure 28-2

Removing Medication from Ampule

Goal: To safely withdraw prescribed drug dose from an ampule.

Excellent	Satisfactory	Needs Practice		COMMENTS
___	___	___	1. Gather equipment. Check medication order against original physician's order according to agency policy.	
___	___	___	2. Wash your hands.	
___	___	___	3. Tap ampule stem or twist your wrist quickly while holding ampule vertically.	
___	___	___	4. Wrap small gauze pad or dry alcohol swab around neck of ampule.	
___	___	___	5. Use a snapping motion to break off top of ampule along the prescored line at its neck. Always break away from your body.	
___	___	___	6. Remove cap from needle by pulling it straight off. Insert needle into ampule, being careful not to touch the rim. (Some agencies recommend the use of a filter needle when withdrawing solution from an ampule.)	
___	___	___	7. Withdraw medication in the amount ordered. Do not inject air into solutions. Use either of the following methods:	
___	___	___	a. Insert tip of needle into ampule, which is *upright* on a flat surface and withdraw fluid into syringe. Touch plunger at knob only.	
___	___	___	b. Insert tip of needle into ampule and *invert* ampule. Keep needle centered and not touching sides of ampule. Remove prescribed amount of medication. Touch plunger at knob only.	
___	___	___	8. Do not expel any air bubbles that may form in the solution. Wait until needle has been withdrawn to tap syringe and expel air carefully. Check amount of medication in syringe and discard any surplus.	

Procedure 28-2

Removing Medication
from Ampule (continued)

Goal: To safely withdraw prescribed drug dose
from an ampule.

COMMENTS

Excellent	Satisfactory	Needs Practice		
___	___	___	9. Discard ampule in a suitable container after comparing with medication card or Kardex.	
___	___	___	10. Replace cap carefully over needle on syringe.	
___	___	___	11. Wash your hands.	

Procedure Checklists to Accompany Taylor Fundamentals of Nursing: The Art and Science of Nursing Care, 4th Edition

Name _____   Date _____

Unit _____   Position _____

Instructor/Evaluator _____   Position _____

Excellent ▼	Satisfactory ▼	Needs Practice ▼	**Procedure 28-3** **Removing Medication from Vial** **Goal:** To safely withdraw prescribed drug dose from vial.	COMMENTS
——	——	——	1. Gather equipment. Check medication order against original physician's order according to agency policy.	
——	——	——	2. Wash your hands.	
——	——	——	3. Remove metal or plastic cap on vial that protects rubber stopper.	
——	——	——	4. Swab rubber top with alcohol swab.	
——	——	——	5. Remove cap from needle by pulling it straight off. (Some agencies recommend use of a filter needle when withdrawing premixed medications from multidose vials.) Draw back an amount of air into syringe equal to specific dose of medication to be withdrawn.	
——	——	——	6. Pierce rubber stopper in the center with the needle tip and inject measured air into the space above the solution. (Do not inject air into the solution.) Vial may be positioned upright on a flat surface or inverted.	
——	——	——	7. Invert vial and withdraw needle tip slightly so that it is below the fluid level.	
——	——	——	8. Draw up prescribed amount of medication while holding syringe at eye level and vertically. Be careful to touch the plunger at knob only.	
——	——	——	9. If any air bubbles accumulate in syringe, tap syringe barrel sharply and move needle past fluid into the air space to reinject the air bubble into vial. Return needle tip to the solution and continue withdrawal of medication.	
——	——	——	10. After correct dose is withdrawn, remove needle from vial and carefully replace cap over needle.	
——	——	——	11. If using a multidose vial, store vial containing remaining medication according to agency policy.	
——	——	——	12. Wash your hands.	

Procedure Checklists to Accompany Taylor Fundamentals of Nursing: The Art and Science of Nursing Care, 4ᵗʰ Edition

Name _____ Date _____

Unit _____ Position _____

Instructor/Evaluator _____ Position _____

Excellent ▼	Satisfactory ▼	Needs Practice ▼	

Procedure 28-4

Mixing Insulins in One Syringe

Goal: To safely withdraw prescribed insulin doses from two vials into one syringe.

COMMENTS

Excellent	Satisfactory	Needs Practice	
____	____	____	1. Gather equipment. Check medication order against original physician's order according to agency policy.
____	____	____	2. Wash your hands.
____	____	____	3. If necessary, remove metal cap that protects rubber stopper on each vial.
____	____	____	4. If insulin is a suspension (NPH, lente), shake vial vigorously.
____	____	____	5. Cleanse rubber tops with alcohol swabs.
____	____	____	6. Remove cap from needle. Inject air into the modified insulin preparation (e.g., NPH insulin). Touch plunger at knob only. Use an amount of air equal to the amount of medication to be withdrawn. Do not allow needle to touch medication in the vial. Remove needle.
____	____	____	7. Inject air into the clear insulin without additional protein (e.g., regular insulin). Use an amount of air equal to the amount of medication to be withdrawn. Do not bubble the air through the medication.
____	____	____	8. Invert vial of clear insulin and aspirate the amount prescribed. Remove needle from vial.
____	____	____	9. Cleanse rubber top of the modified insulin vial. Insert needle into this vial, invert it, and withdraw medication. Carefully replace cap over needle.
____	____	____	10. Store vials according to agency recommendations.
____	____	____	11. Wash your hands.

Procedure Checklists to Accompany Taylor Fundamentals of Nursing: The Art and Science of Nursing Care, 4ᵗʰ Edition

Name _____ Date _____

Unit _____ Position _____

Instructor/Evaluator _____ Position _____

Procedure 28-5

Administering an Intradermal Injection

Goal: To safely deliver prescribed drug dose to area just below the epidermis.

Excellent	Satisfactory	Needs Practice		COMMENTS
▼	▼	▼		
——	——	——	1. Assemble equipment and check physician's order.	
——	——	——	2. Explain procedure to patient.	
——	——	——	3. Wash your hands. Don disposable gloves (optional).	
——	——	——	4. If necessary, withdraw medication from ampule or vial as described in Procedures 28-2 and 28-3.	
——	——	——	5. Select area on inner aspect of forearm that is not heavily pigmented or covered with hair. Upper chest or upper back beneath the scapulae also are sites for intradermal injections.	
——	——	——	6. Cleanse area with alcohol swab by wiping with a firm, circular motion and moving outward from the injection site. Allow skin to dry. If skin is oily, clean area with pledget moistened with acetone.	
——	——	——	7. Use nondominant hand to spread skin taut over injection site.	
——	——	——	8. Remove needle cap with nondominant hand by pulling it straight off.	
——	——	——	9. Place needle almost flat against patient's skin, bevel side up. Insert needle into skin so that point of needle can be seen through skin. Insert needle only about 1/8 inch.	
——	——	——	10. Slowly inject agent while watching for a small wheal or blister to appear. If none appears, withdraw needle slightly.	
——	——	——	11. Withdraw needle quickly at the same angle it was inserted.	
——	——	——	12. Do not massage area after removing needle.	
——	——	——	13. Do not recap used needle. Discard needle and syringe in the appropriate receptacle.	
——	——	——	14. Assist patient into a position of comfort.	

Excellent ▼	Satisfactory ▼	Needs Practice ▼	

Procedure 28-5

Administering an
Intradermal Injection (continued)

Goal: To safely deliver prescribed drug dose
to area just below the epidermis.

COMMENTS

Excellent	Satisfactory	Needs Practice		
——	——	——	15. Remove gloves, if worn, and dispose of them properly. Wash your hands.	
——	——	——	16. Chart administration of medication.	
——	——	——	17. Observe area for signs of a reaction at ordered intervals, usually 24–72-hour periods. Inform patient of this inspection. In some agencies, a circle may be drawn on the skin around injection site.	

Procedure Checklists to Accompany Taylor Fundamentals of Nursing: The Art and Science of Nursing Care, 4th Edition

Name _____   Date _____

Unit _____   Position _____

Instructor/Evaluator _____   Position _____

Procedure 28-6

Administering a Subcutaneous Injection

Goal: To safely deliver prescribed drug dose into subcutaneous tissue.

Excellent	Satisfactory	Needs Practice		COMMENTS
▼	▼	▼		
____	____	____	1. Assemble equipment and check physician's order.	
____	____	____	2. Explain procedure to patient.	
____	____	____	3. Wash your hands.	
____	____	____	4. If necessary, withdraw medication from ampule or vial as described in Procedures 28-2 and 28-3.	
____	____	____	5. Identify patient carefully. See Procedure 28-1, Action 12. Close curtain to provide privacy. Don disposable gloves (optional).	
____	____	____	6. Have patient assume a position appropriate for the most commonly used sites:	
____	____	____	a. Outer aspect of upper arm—Patient's arm should be relaxed and at side of body.	
____	____	____	b. Abdomen—Patient may lie in a semirecumbent position.	
____	____	____	c. Anterior thighs—Patient may sit or lie with leg relaxed.	
____	____	____	7. Locate site of choice according to directions given in this chapter. Ensure that area is not tender and is free of lumps or nodules.	
____	____	____	8. Clean area around injection site with an alcohol swab. Use a firm, circular motion while moving outward from the injection site. Allow antiseptic to dry. Leave alcohol swab in a clean area for reuse when withdrawing the needle.	
____	____	____	9. Remove needle cap with nondominant hand, pulling it straight off.	
____	____	____	10. Grasp and bunch area surrounding injection site or spread skin at site.	

Procedure 28-6

Administering a Subcutaneous Injection (continued)

Goal: To safely deliver prescribed drug dose into subcutaneous tissue.

Excellent	Satisfactory	Needs Practice		COMMENTS
▼	▼	▼		
___	___	___	11. Hold syringe in dominant hand between thumb and forefinger. Inject needle quickly at an angle of 45–90°, depending on amount and turgor of tissue and length of needle, as shown.	
___	___	___	12. After needle is in place, release tissue and immediately move your nondominant hand to steady lower end of syringe. Slide your dominant hand to tip of barrel.	
___	___	___	13. Aspirate, if recommended, by pulling back gently on syringe plunger to determine if needle is in a blood vessel (optional). If blood appears, needle should be withdrawn and the medication, syringe, and needle discarded. Prepare a new syringe with new medication. *Do not aspirate when giving insulin or heparin.*	
___	___	___	14. If no blood appears, inject solution slowly.	
___	___	___	15. Withdraw needle quickly at the same angle at which it was inserted, as shown.	
___	___	___	16. Massage area gently with alcohol swab. (Do not massage a subcutaneous heparin or insulin injection site.)	
___	___	___	17. Do not recap used needle. Discard needle and syringe in appropriate receptacle.	
___	___	___	18. Assist patient to a position of comfort.	
___	___	___	19. Remove gloves, if worn, and dispose of them properly. Wash your hands.	
___	___	___	20. Chart administration of medication.	
___	___	___	21. Evaluate patient response to medication within an appropriate time frame.	

Procedure Checklists to Accompany Taylor Fundamentals of Nursing: The Art and Science of Nursing Care, 4th Edition

Name _____   Date _____

Unit _____   Position _____

Instructor/Evaluator _____   Position _____

Procedure 28-7

Administering an Intramuscular Injection

Goal: To safely deliver prescribed drug dose into muscle tissue.

Excellent	Satisfactory	Needs Practice		COMMENTS
____	____	____	1. Assemble equipment and check physician's order.	
____	____	____	2. Explain procedure to patient.	
____	____	____	3. Wash your hands.	
____	____	____	4. If necessary, withdraw medication from ampule or vial as described in Procedures 28-2 and 28-3.	
____	____	____	5. Do not add air to syringe.	
____	____	____	6. Provide for privacy. Have patient assume a position for the site selected.	
____	____	____	a. Ventrogluteal—Patient may lie on back or side with hip and knee flexed.	
____	____	____	b. Vastus lateralis—Patient may lie on the back or may assume a sitting position.	
____	____	____	c. Deltoid—Patient may sit or lie with arm relaxed.	
____	____	____	d. Dorsogluteal—Patient may lie prone with toes pointing inward or on side with upper leg flexed and placed in front of lower leg.	
____	____	____	7. Locate site of choice according to directions given in this chapter and ensure that the area is not tender and is free of lumps or nodules. Don disposable gloves (optional).	
____	____	____	8. Clean area thoroughly with alcohol swab, using friction. Allow alcohol to dry.	
____	____	____	9. Remove needle cap by pulling it straight off.	
____	____	____	10. Displace skin in a Z-track manner or spread skin at the site using your nondominant hand.	

Administering an Intramuscular Injection (continued)

Goal: To safely deliver prescribed drug dose into muscle tissue.

Excellent	Satisfactory	Needs Practice		COMMENTS
✓			11. Hold syringe in your dominant hand between thumb and forefinger. Quickly dart needle into the tissue at a 90° angle.	
✓			12. As soon as needle is in place, move your nondominant hand to hold lower end of syringe. Slide your dominant hand to tip of barrel.	
✓			13. Aspirate by slowly (for at least 5 seconds) pulling back on plunger to determine whether or not needle is in a blood vessel. If blood is aspirated, discard needle, syringe, and medication. Prepare a new sterile setup and inject in another site.	
✓			14. If no blood is aspirated, inject solution slowly (10 seconds per mL of medication).	
	✓		15. Remove needle slowly and steadily. Release displaced tissue if Z-track technique was used.	
✓			16. Apply gentle pressure at site with a small, dry sponge.	
✓			17. Do not recap used needle. Discard needle and syringe in appropriate receptacle.	
✓			18. Assist patient to a position of comfort. Encourage patient to exercise leg if possible.	
✓			19. Remove gloves, if worn, and dispose of them properly. Wash your hands.	
✓			20. Chart administration of medication.	
✓			21. Evaluate patient response to medication within an appropriate time frame. Assess site, if possible, within 2–4 hours after administration.	

Procedure Checklists to Accompany Taylor Fundamentals of Nursing: The Art and Science of Nursing Care, 4ᵗʰ Edition

Name _____ Date _____

Unit _____ Position _____

Instructor/Evaluator _____ Position _____

Procedure 28-8

Adding Medications to an IV Solution

Goal: To safely introduce prescribed drug dose into an IV solution.

Excellent	Satisfactory	Needs Practice		COMMENTS
▼	▼	▼		
___	___	___	1. Gather all equipment and bring to patient's bedside. Check medication order against physician's order.	
___	___	___	2. Explain procedure to patient.	
___	___	___	3. Wash your hands.	
___	___	___	4. Identify patient by checking the band on the patient's wrist and asking patient his/her name.	
___	___	___	5. Add medications to IV solution that is infusing:	
___	___	___	a. Check that volume in bag or bottle is adequate.	
___	___	___	b. Close IV clamp.	
___	___	___	c. Clean medication port with alcohol swab.	
___	___	___	d. Steady container. Uncap needle or needleless device and insert it into port. Inject medication.	
___	___	___	e. Remove container from IV pole and gently rotate solution.	
___	___	___	f. Rehang container, open clamp, and readjust flow rate.	
___	___	___	g. Attach label to container so that dose of added medication is apparent.	
___	___	___	6. Add medication to IV solution before infusion:	
___	___	___	a. Carefully remove any protective cover and locate injection port. Clean with alcohol swab.	
___	___	___	b. Uncap needle or needleless device and insert into port. Inject medication.	
___	___	___	c. Withdraw needle and insert spike into proper entry site on bag or bottle.	

Procedure 28-8

Adding Medications
to an IV Solution (continued)

Excellent ▼	Satisfactory ▼	Needs Practice ▼		COMMENTS
			Goal: To safely introduce prescribed drug dose into an IV solution.	
——	——	——	d. With tubing clamped, gently rotate IV solution in the bag or bottle. Hang IV.	
——	——	——	e. Attach label to container so that dose of added medication is apparent.	
——	——	——	7. Dispose of equipment according to agency policy.	
——	——	——	8. Wash your hands.	
——	——	——	9. Chart addition of medication to IV solution.	
——	——	——	10. Evaluate patient's response to medication within appropriate time frame.	

Procedure Checklists to Accompany Taylor Fundamentals of Nursing: The Art and Science of Nursing Care, 4th Edition

Name _____   Date _____

Unit _____   Position _____

Instructor/Evaluator _____   Position _____

Procedure 28-9

Adding Bolus IV Medication to an Existing IV

Goal: To safely introduce prescribed drug dose directly into intravenous line.

Excellent	Satisfactory	Needs Practice		COMMENTS
___	___	___	1. Gather equipment and bring to patient's bedside. Check medication order against physician's order. Check a drug resource to clarify if medication needs to be diluted before administration.	
___	___	___	2. Explain procedure to patient.	
___	___	___	3. Wash your hands. Don clean gloves.	
___	___	___	4. Identify patient by checking the band on the patient's wrist and asking patient his/her name.	
___	___	___	5. Assess IV site for presence of inflammation or infiltration.	
___	___	___	6. Select injection port on tubing closest to the venipuncture site. Clean port with alcohol swab.	
___	___	___	7. Uncap syringe. Steady port with your nondominant hand while inserting needleless device or needle into the center of port.	
___	___	___	8. Move your nondominant hand to the section of IV tubing just beyond injection port. Fold tubing between your fingers to temporarily stop the flow of IV solution.	
___	___	___	9. Pull back slightly on plunger just until blood appears in tubing.	
___	___	___	10. Inject medication at the prescribed rate.	
___	___	___	11. Remove needle. Do not cap it. Release tubing and allow IV to flow at the proper rate.	
___	___	___	12. Dispose of syringe in proper receptacle.	
___	___	___	13. Remove gloves and wash your hands.	
___	___	___	14. Chart administration of medication.	
___	___	___	15. Evaluate patient's response to medication within appropriate time frame.	

Procedure Checklists to Accompany Taylor Fundamentals of Nursing: The Art and Science of Nursing Care, 4th Edition

Name _____ Date _____

Unit _____ Position _____

Instructor/Evaluator _____ Position _____

Procedure 28-10

Administering IV Medications by Piggyback, Volume Control Administration Set, or Mini-infusion Pump

Goal: To safely deliver prescribed drug dose by intravenous infusion over a short period at the prescribed interval.

Excellent ▼	Satisfactory ▼	Needs Practice ▼		COMMENTS
___	___	___	1. Gather all equipment and bring to patient's bedside. Check medication order against original physician's order according to agency policy.	
___	___	___	2. Identify patient by checking the identification band on patient's wrist and asking patient his or her name.	
___	___	___	3. Explain procedure to patient.	
___	___	___	4. Wash your hands and don gloves.	
___	___	___	5. Assess IV site for presence of inflammation or infiltration.	
			For Piggyback Infusion	
___	___	___	6. Attach infusion tubing to the piggyback set containing diluted medication. Place label on tubing with appropriate date and attach needle or needleless device to end of tubing according to manufacturer's directions. Open clamp and prime tubing. (See Action 4, Procedure 45-1.) Close clamp.	
___	___	___	7. Hang piggyback container on IV pole, positioning it higher than the primary IV according to manufacturer's recommendations. Use metal or plastic hook to lower primary IV.	
___	___	___	8. Use alcohol swab to clean appropriate port.	
___	___	___	9. Connect piggyback setup to either:	
___	___	___	a. Needleless port	
___	___	___	b. Stopcock: Turn stopcock to open position.	

Procedure 28-10

Administering IV Medications by Piggyback, Volume Control Administration Set, or Mini-infusion Pump (continued)

Goal: To safely deliver prescribed drug dose by intravenous infusion over a short period at the prescribed interval.

Excellent ▼	Satisfactory ▼	Needs Practice ▼		COMMENTS
___	___	___	c. Primary IV line: Uncap needle and insert into secondary IV port closest to the top of the primary tubing. Use a strip of tape to secure secondary set tubing to primary infusion tubing. Primary line is left unclamped if port has a back-flow valve.	
___	___	___	10. Open clamp on piggyback set and regulate flow at the prescribed delivery rate or set rate for secondary infusion on infusion pump. Monitor medication infusion at periodic intervals.	
___	___	___	11. Clamp tubing on piggyback set when solution is infused. Follow agency policy regarding disposal of equipment.	
___	___	___	12. Readjust flow rate of the primary IV.	
			Using a Mini-infusion Pump	
___	___	___	13. Connect prepared syringe to mini-infusion tubing.	
___	___	___	14. Fill tubing with medication by applying gentle pressure to syringe plunger.	
___	___	___	15. Insert syringe into mini-infuser pump as per manufacturer's directions.	
___	___	___	16. Connect mini-infusion tubing to appropriate connector as in Action 9.	
___	___	___	17. Program pump to begin infusion. Set alarm if recommended by manufacturer.	
___	___	___	18. Recheck flow rate of primary IV once pump has completed delivery of medication.	
			Using a Volume Control Administration Set	
___	___	___	19. Withdraw medication from vial or ampule into prepared syringe. See Procedure 28-2 or 28-3.	
___	___	___	20. Open clamp between IV solution and the volume-control administration set or secondary setup. Follow manufacturer's instructions and fill with desired amount of IV solution. Close clamp.	
___	___	___	21. Use an alcohol swab to clean injection port on the secondary setup.	

Procedure 28-10

Administering IV Medications by Piggyback, Volume Control Administration Set, or Mini-infusion Pump (continued)

Goal: To safely deliver prescribed drug dose by intravenous infusion over a short period at the prescribed interval.

Excellent	Satisfactory	Needs Practice		COMMENTS
▼	▼	▼		
___	___	___	22. Remove cap and insert needle or blunt needleless device into port while holding syringe steady. Inject medication. Mix gently with IV solution.	
___	___	___	23. Open clamp below the secondary setup and regulate at prescribed delivery rate. Monitor medication infusion at periodic intervals.	
___	___	___	24. Attach label to volume-control device.	
___	___	___	25. Place syringe with uncapped needle in designated container.	
___	___	___	26. Wash your hands.	
___	___	___	27. Chart administration of medication after it has been infused.	
___	___	___	28. Evaluate patient's response to medication within appropriate time frame.	

Procedure Checklists to Accompany Taylor Fundamentals of Nursing: The Art and Science of Nursing Care, 4th Edition

Name _____   Date _____

Unit _____   Position _____

Instructor/Evaluator _____   Position _____

Procedure 28-11

Introducing Drugs Through a Heparin or Intravenous Lock Using Saline Flush

Goal: To safely deliver prescribed drug dose by intravenous infusion over a short period at the prescribed interval into a heparin or intravenous lock device.

Excellent	Satisfactory	Needs Practice		COMMENTS
▼	▼	▼		
——	——	——	1. Assemble equipment and check physician's order.	
——	——	——	2. Explain procedure to patient.	
——	——	——	3. Wash your hands.	
——	——	——	4. Withdraw 1–2 mL of sterile saline from vial into syringe as described in Procedure 28-3.	
——	——	——	5. Don clean gloves.	
——	——	——	6. Administer medication.	
			For Bolus IV Injection:	
——	——	——	a. Check drug package for correct injection rate for the IV push route.	
——	——	——	b. Clean port of the lock with alcohol swab.	
——	——	——	c. Stabilize port with your nondominant hand and insert needleless device or needle of syringe of normal saline into the port.	
——	——	——	d. Aspirate gently and check for blood return. (Blood return does not always occur even though lock is patent.)	
——	——	——	e. Gently flush with 1 mL of normal saline. Remove syringe.	
——	——	——	f. Insert blunt needleless device or needle of syringe with medication into port and gently inject medication, using a watch to verify correct injection rate. Do not force the injection if there is resistance. If lock is clogged, it has to be changed. Remove medication syringe and needle when administration is completed.	

Procedure 28-11

Introducing Drugs Through a Heparin or Intravenous Lock Using Saline Flush (continued)

Excellent ▼	Satisfactory ▼	Needs Practice ▼	

Goal: To safely deliver prescribed drug dose by intravenous infusion over a short period at the prescribed interval into a heparin or intravenous lock device.

COMMENTS

For Administration of a Drug by Way of an Intermittent Delivery System:

___ ___ ___   a. Use a drug resource book to check correct flow rate of medication. (Usual rate is 30–60 minutes).

___ ___ ___   b. Connect infusion tubing to the medication setup according to manufacturer's directions. Hang IV setup on a pole. Open clamp and allow solution to clear IV tubing of air. Reclamp tubing.

___ ___ ___   c. Attach needleless connector or sterile 25-gauge needle to end of infusion tubing.

___ ___ ___   d. Clean port of the lock with alcohol swab.

___ ___ ___   e. Stabilize port with your nondominant hand and insert needleless device or needle of syringe of normal saline into the port.

___ ___ ___   f. Aspirate gently and check for blood return. (Blood return does not always occur even though lock is patent.)

___ ___ ___   g. Gently flush with 1 mL of normal saline. Remove syringe.

___ ___ ___   h. Insert blunt needleless device or needle attached to tubing into port. If necessary, secure with tape.

___ ___ ___   i. Open clamp and regulate flow rate or attach to IV pump or controller according to manufacturer's directions. Close clamp when infusion is complete.

Procedure 28-11

Introducing Drugs Through a Heparin or Intravenous Lock Using Saline Flush (continued)

Goal: To safely deliver prescribed drug dose by intravenous infusion over a short period at the prescribed interval into a heparin or intravenous lock device.

Excellent	Satisfactory	Needs Practice		COMMENTS
▼	▼	▼		
——	——	——	j. Remove the needleless connector or needle from lock. Carefully replace uncapped used needle or needleless device with a new sterile one. Allow medication setup to hang on the pole for future use according to agency policy.	
			Stabilize port with your nondominant hand and insert needleless device or needle of syringe of normal saline into the port.	
			Flush reservoir with 1 to 2 mL of sterile saline. Remove syringe and discard in appropriate receptacle. Remove gloves and discard appropriately.	
——	——	——	7. Wash your hands.	
——	——	——	8. Injection site and IV lock should be checked at least every 8 hours and a small amount of saline administered if medication is not given at least that often.	
——	——	——	9. Heparin lock should be changed at least every 48 hours or according to agency policy. A clogged lock should be changed immediately.	
——	——	——	10. Chart administration of medication or saline flush.	

Procedure Checklists to Accompany Taylor Fundamentals of Nursing: The Art and Science of Nursing Care, 4th Edition

Name _____   Date _____

Unit _____   Position _____

Instructor/Evaluator _____   Position _____

Procedure 28-12

Administering an Eye Irrigation

Goal: To safely remove secretions from eye.

Excellent	Satisfactory	Needs Practice		COMMENTS
▼	▼	▼		
___	___	___	1. Explain procedure to patient.	
___	___	___	2. Assemble equipment.	
___	___	___	3. Wash your hands.	
___	___	___	4. Have patient sit or lie with head tilted toward the side of the affected eye. Protect patient and bed with a waterproof pad.	
___	___	___	5. Don disposable gloves. Clean lids and lashes with cotton ball moistened with normal saline or solution ordered for irrigation. Wipe from inner canthus to outer canthus. Discard cotton ball after each wipe.	
___	___	___	6. Place curved basin at the cheek on the side of affected eye to receive irrigating solution. If patient is sitting up, ask him/her to support basin.	
___	___	___	7. Expose lower conjunctival sac and hold upper lid open with your nondominant hand.	
___	___	___	8. Hold irrigator about 2.5 cm (1 inch) from eye. Direct flow of solution from the inner to the outer canthus along the conjunctival sac.	
___	___	___	9. Irrigate until solution is clear or all solution has been used. Use only sufficient force to gently remove secretions from conjunctiva. Avoid touching any part of eye with irrigating tip.	
___	___	___	10. Have patient close eye periodically during procedure.	
___	___	___	11. After irrigation, dry area with cotton balls or gauze sponge. Offer towel to patient if face and neck are wet.	
___	___	___	12. Remove gloves and wash your hands.	
___	___	___	13. Chart irrigation, appearance of eye, drainage, and patient's response.	

Procedure Checklists to Accompany Taylor Fundamentals of Nursing: The Art and Science of Nursing Care, 4th Edition

Name _____ Date _____

Unit _____ Position _____

Instructor/Evaluator _____ Position _____

Procedure 28-13

Administering an Ear Irrigation

Goal: To safely cleanse external auditory canal.

Excellent	Satisfactory	Needs Practice		COMMENTS
▼	▼	▼		
——	——	——	1. Explain procedure to patient.	
——	——	——	2. Assemble equipment. Protect patient and bed linens with a moisture-proof pad.	
——	——	——	3. Wash your hands.	
——	——	——	4. Have patient sit up or lie with head tilted toward the side of the affected ear. Have patient support a basin under the ear to receive the irrigating solution.	
——	——	——	5. Clean pinna and meatus at the auditory canal as necessary with applicators dipped in normal saline or irrigating solution.	
——	——	——	6. Fill bulb syringe with solution. If using an irrigating container, allow air to escape from tubing.	
——	——	——	7. Straighten auditory canal by pulling the pinna down and back for an infant and up and back for an adult.	
——	——	——	8. Direct a steady, slow stream of solution against roof of auditory canal, using only sufficient force to remove secretions. Do not occlude auditory canal with irrigating nozzle. Allow solution to flow out unimpeded.	
——	——	——	9. When irrigation is complete, place cotton ball loosely in the auditory meatus and have patient lie on the side of the affected ear on a towel or absorbent pad.	
——	——	——	10. Wash your hands.	
——	——	——	11. Chart irrigation, appearance of drainage, and patient's response.	
——	——	——	12. Return in 10–15 minutes and remove cotton ball and assess drainage.	

Procedure Checklists to Accompany Taylor Fundamentals of Nursing: The Art and Science of Nursing Care, 4th Edition

Name _____ Date _____

Unit _____ Position _____

Instructor/Evaluator _____ Position _____

Procedure 29-1

Preoperative Patient Care: Hospitalized Patient

Goal: To provide the necessary physical and psychological preparation for surgery.

Excellent	Satisfactory	Needs Practice		COMMENTS
✓	—	—	1. Identify patients for whom surgery is a greater risk:	
✓	—	—	a. Very young or elderly patients.	
✓	—	—	b. Obese or malnourished patients.	
✓	—	—	c. Patients with fluid and electrolyte imbalances.	
✓	—	—	d. Patients in poor general health from chronic diseases and infectious processes.	
—	—	—	e. Patients taking certain medications (i.e., anticoagulants, antibiotics, diuretics, depressants, steroids).	
—	—	—	f. Patients who are extremely anxious.	
✓	—	—	2. Review nursing database, history, and physical examination. Check that baseline data are recorded; report those that are abnormal.	
✓	—	—	3. Check that diagnostic testing has been completed and results are available; identify and report abnormal results.	
✓	—	—	4. Promote optimal nutritional and hydration status.	
✓	—	—	5. Identify learning needs of patient and family. Conduct preoperative teaching regarding the following:	
✓	—	—	a. Coughing and deep-breathing exercises; respiratory therapy regimes.	
✓	—	—	b. Pain management after surgery.	
—	—	✓	c. Leg exercises and early ambulation.	
—	✓	—	d. Postoperative equipment and monitoring devices.	
—	✓	—	e. Home care requirements.	

Procedure 29-1

Preoperative Patient Care: Hospitalized Patient (continued)

Goal: To provide the necessary physical and psychological preparation for surgery.

Excellent	Satisfactory	Needs Practice		COMMENTS

Day Before Surgery:

6. Provide emotional support. Answer questions realistically. Provide spiritual guidance if requested. Include family when possible.

7. Follow preoperative fluid and food restrictions.

8. Prepare for elimination needs during and after surgery.

9. Attend to patient's special hygiene needs (e.g., use of antiseptic cleaning agents to prepare surgical site).

10. Provide for adequate rest.

Day of Surgery:

11. Check that proper identification band is on patient.

12. Check that preoperative consent forms are signed, witnessed, and correct and that advanced directives are in the medical record (as applicable), and medical record is in order.

13. Check vital signs. Notify physician of any pertinent changes (e.g., rise or drop in blood pressure, elevated temperature, cough, symptoms of infection).

14. Provide hygiene and oral care. Remind patient of food and fluid restrictions and time when NPO for surgery.

15. Continue nutritional and hydration preparation.

16. Remove cosmetics and prostheses (e.g., contact lenses, false eyelashes, denture, and so forth). Assess for loose teeth.

17. Have patient empty bladder and bowel before surgery.

18. Place valuables in appropriate area. Hospital safe is most appropriate place for valuables. They should not be placed in narcotics drawer.

19. Attend to any special preoperative orders.

20. Complete preoperative checklist and record patient's preoperative preparation.

21. Administer preoperative medication as prescribed by physician/anesthesia provider.

Procedure Checklists to Accompany Taylor Fundamentals of Nursing: The Art and Science of Nursing Care, 4ᵗʰ Edition

Name _____ Date _____

Unit _____ Position _____

Instructor/Evaluator _____ Position _____

Excellent	Satisfactory	Needs Practice	*Procedure 29-2* **Postoperative Care When Patient Returns to Room** **Goal:** To provide the necessary physical and psychological care following surgery.	COMMENTS
▼	▼	▼		
			Immediate	
___	___	___	1. Place patient in safe position (high Fowler's or side-lying). Note level of consciousness.	
___	___	___	2. Monitor and record vital signs frequently. Assessment order may vary, but usual frequency includes taking vital signs every 15 minutes the first hour, every 30 minutes the next 2 hours, every hour for 4 hours, and finally, every 4 hours.	
___	___	___	3. Provide for warmth. Assess skin color and condition.	
___	___	___	4. Check dressings for color, odor, and amount of drainage. Feel under patient for bleeding.	
___	___	___	5. Verify that all tubes and drains are patent and equipment is operative. Note amount of drainage in collection device.	
___	___	___	6. Maintain intravenous infusion at correct rate.	
___	___	___	7. Provide for a safe environment. Keep bed in low position with side rails up. Have call bell within patient's reach.	
___	___	___	8. Relieve pain by administering medications ordered by physician. Check record to verify if analgesic medication was administered in PACU.	
___	___	___	9. Record assessments and interventions on chart.	
			General	
___	___	___	10. Promote optimal respiratory function:	
___	___	___	a. Coughing and deep breathing.	
___	___	___	b. Incentive spirometry.	
___	___	___	c. Early ambulation.	

Procedure 29-2

Postoperative Care When Patient Returns to Room (continued)

Goal: To provide the necessary physical and psychological care following surgery.

Excellent	Satisfactory	Needs Practice		COMMENTS
▼	▼	▼		
—	—	—	d. Frequent position change.	
—	—	—	e. Administration of oxygen as ordered.	
—	—	—	11. Maintain adequate circulation:	
—	—	—	a. Frequent position changes.	
—	—	—	b. Early ambulation.	
—	—	—	c. Application of antiembolic stockings or pneumatic compression devices if ordered by physician.	
—	—	—	d. Leg and range-of-motion exercises if not contraindicated.	
—	—	—	12. Assess urinary elimination status:	
—	—	—	a. Promote voiding by offering bedpan at regular intervals.	
—	—	—	b. Monitor catheter drainage if present.	
—	—	—	c. Measure intake and output.	
—	—	—	13. Promote optimal nutrition status and return of gastrointestinal function:	
—	—	—	a. Assess for return of peristalsis.	
—	—	—	b. Assist with diet progression.	
—	—	—	c. Encourage fluid intake.	
—	—	—	d. Monitor intake.	
—	—	—	e. Medicate for nausea and vomiting as ordered by physician.	
—	—	—	14. Promote wound healing:	
—	—	—	a. Use surgical asepsis.	
—	—	—	b. Assess condition of wound.	
—	—	—	c. Assess any drainage.	
—	—	—	15. Provide for rest and comfort.	
—	—	—	16. Provide emotional and spiritual support.	

Procedure Checklists to Accompany Taylor Fundamentals of Nursing: The Art and Science of Nursing Care, 4ᵗʰ Edition

Name _____ Date _____

Unit _____ Position _____

Instructor/Evaluator _____ Position _____

Excellent	Satisfactory	Needs Practice	*Procedure 36-1* **Giving a Bed Bath**	COMMENTS
▼	▼	▼	**Goal:** To provide or assist with personal hygiene.	
___	___	___	1. Discuss procedure with patient and assess patient's ability to assist in the bathing process as well as personal hygiene preferences. Review patient's chart for any limitations in physical activity.	
___	___	___	2. Bring necessary equipment to bedside stand or overbed table. Remove sequential compression devices and antiembolism stockings from lower extremities according to agency protocol.	
___	___	___	3. Close curtains around bed and close door to the room if possible.	
___	___	___	4. Offer patient a bedpan or urinal.	
___	___	___	5. Wash your hands.	
___	___	___	6. Raise patient's bed to the high position.	
___	___	___	7. Lower the side rails nearer to you and assist patient to the side of the bed where you will work. Have patient lie on his/her back.	
___	___	___	8. Loosen top covers and remove all except top sheet. Place bath blanket over patient and then remove top sheet while patient holds bath blanket in place. If linen is to be reused, fold it over a chair. Place soiled linen in laundry bag.	
___	___	___	9. Assist patient with oral hygiene, as necessary, and as described in Procedure 36-5.	
___	___	___	10. Remove patient's gown and keep bath blanket in place. If patient has an intravenous line and is not wearing a gown with snap sleeves, remove gown from other arm first. Lower intravenous container and pass gown over tubing and container. Rehang container and check drip rate.	

Procedure 36-1

Giving a Bed Bath (continued)

Excellent ▼	Satisfactory ▼	Needs Practice ▼	
			Goal: To provide or assist with personal hygiene. COMMENTS
——	——	——	11. Raise side rail. Fill basin with a sufficient amount of comfortably warm (43–46° C [110–115° F]) water. Change as necessary throughout the bath. Lower side rail closer to you when you return to the bedside to begin the bath.
——	——	——	12. Fold washcloth like a mitt on your hand so there are no loose ends (as illustrated).
——	——	——	13. Lay towel across patient's chest and on top of bath blanket.
——	——	——	14. With no soap on the washcloth, wipe one eye from inner part of the eye near the nose to the outer part. Rinse or turn cloth before washing other eye.
——	——	——	15. Bathe patient's face, neck, and ears, avoiding soap on the face if the patient prefers.
——	——	——	16. Expose patient's far arm and place towel lengthwise under it. Using firm strokes, wash arm and axilla, rinse, and dry.
——	——	——	17. Place folded towel on bed next to patient's hand and put basin on towel. Soak patient's hand in basin. Wash, rinse, and dry hand.
——	——	——	18. Repeat Actions 16 and 17 for the arm near to you. (An option for a shorter nurse or one prone to back strain might be to bathe one side of patient and move to the other side of bed to complete the bath.)
——	——	——	19. Spread towel across patient's chest. Lower bath blanket to patient's umbilical area. Wash, rinse, and dry patient's chest. Keep patient's chest covered with towel between the wash and rinse. Pay special attention to skin folds under patient's breasts.
——	——	——	20. Lower bath blanket to patient's perineal area. Place towel over patient's chest.
——	——	——	21. Wash, rinse, and dry patient's abdomen. Carefully inspect and cleanse umbilical area and any abdominal folds or creases.
——	——	——	22. Return bath blanket to original position and expose the patient's far leg. Place towel under far leg. Using firm strokes, wash, rinse, and dry patient's leg from ankle to knee and knee to groin.

Procedure 36-1

Giving a Bed Bath (continued)

Excellent	Satisfactory	Needs Practice	**Goal:** To provide or assist with personal hygiene.	**COMMENTS**
▼	▼	▼		
___	___	___	23. Fold towel near patient's foot area and place basin on towel. Place patient's foot in basin while supporting patient's ankle and heel in your hand and leg in your arm. Wash, rinse, and dry, paying particular attention to area between toes.	
___	___	___	24. Repeat Actions 22 and 23 for other leg and foot.	
___	___	___	25. Make sure patient is covered with bath blanket. Change water at this point or earlier if necessary. Assist patient onto his/her side.	
___	___	___	26. Assist patient to a prone or side-lying position. Position bath blanket and towel to expose only back and buttocks.	
___	___	___	27. Wash, rinse, and dry patient's back and buttocks area. Pay particular attention to cleansing between gluteal folds and observe for any indication of redness or skin breakdown in the sacral area.	
___	___	___	28. If not contraindicated, give patient a back rub, as described in Procedure 40-1. Back massage may also be given after perineal care.	
___	___	___	29. Refill basin with clean water. Discard washcloth and towel.	
___	___	___	30. Clean patient's perineal area or set up patient so he/she can complete perineal self-care.	
___	___	___	31. Help patient put on a clean gown and attend to personal hygiene needs.	
___	___	___	32. Protect pillow with a towel and groom patient's hair, as described in text.	
___	___	___	33. Change bed linens, as described in Procedures 36-3 and 36-4.	
___	___	___	34. Record any significant observations and communication on patient's chart.	

Procedure Checklists to Accompany Taylor Fundamentals of Nursing: The Art and Science of Nursing Care, 4ᵗʰ Edition

Name _____ Date _____

Unit _____ Position _____

Instructor/Evaluator _____ Position _____

Excellent ▼	Satisfactory ▼	Needs Practice ▼	**Procedure 36-2** **Applying Antiembolism Stockings** **Goal:** To promote venous return from lower extremities.	COMMENTS
——	——	——	1. Explain the rationale for use of elastic stockings to patient.	
——	——	——	2. Wash your hands.	
——	——	——	3. Assist patient to the supine position. If patient has been sitting or walking, it is necessary to have him/her lie down with legs and feet well elevated for at least 15 minutes before applying stockings.	
——	——	——	4. Provide privacy. Expose legs one at a time and powder lightly unless patient has dry skin. If skin is dry, a lotion may be used. Powders and lotions are not recommended by some manufacturers.	
——	——	——	5. Place hand inside stocking and grasp heel area securely. Turn stocking inside out to the heel area.	
——	——	——	6. Ease foot of stocking over patient's foot and heel. Check that patient's heel is centered in heel pocket of stocking.	
——	——	——	7. Using your fingers and thumbs, carefully grasp edge of stocking and pull it up smoothly over ankle and calf until entire stocking is turned right side out. Pull forward slightly on toe section. Repeat for other leg. Caution patient not to roll stockings partially down.	
——	——	——	8. Wash your hands.	
——	——	——	9. To remove stocking, grasp top of stocking with your thumbs and fingers and smoothly pull stocking off inside out to heel. Support patient's foot and ease stocking over it.	
——	——	——	10. Remove stockings once every shift for 20–30 minutes. Wash and air dry as necessary (according to manufacturer's directions).	
——	——	——	11. Record application of elastic stockings as well as assessment of patient's circulatory status and skin condition.	

Procedure Checklists to Accompany Taylor Fundamentals of Nursing: The Art and Science of Nursing Care, 4th Edition

Name _____ Date _____

Unit _____ Position _____

Instructor/Evaluator _____ Position _____

Excellent	Satisfactory	Needs Practice		COMMENTS
			Procedure 36-3 ## Making an Unoccupied Bed **Goal:** To promote a comfortable bed environment when bed is unoccupied.	
___	___	___	1. Wash your hands.	
___	___	___	2. Assemble equipment and arrange on a bedside chair in the order in which items will be used.	
___	___	___	3. Adjust patient's bed to the high position and drop bed side rails.	
___	___	___	4. Check bed linens for patient's personal items and disconnect call bell or any tubes from bed linens.	
___	___	___	5. Loosen all linen as you move around bed from the head of the bed on the far side to the head of the bed on the near side.	
___	___	___	6. Fold reusable linens, such as sheets, blankets or spread, in place on bed in fourths then hang them over a clean chair.	
___	___	___	7. Snugly roll all soiled linen inside the bottom sheet and place directly into laundry hamper. Do not place them on floor or furniture. Do not hold soiled linens against your uniform.	
___	___	___	8. If possible, shift mattress up to the head of the bed.	
___	___	___	9. Place bottom sheet with its center fold in the center of the bed and high enough to have a sufficient amount of the sheet to tuck under the head of the mattress.	
___	___	___	10. Place drawsheet with its center fold in the center of the bed and position so it will be located under patient's mid-section. If using a protective pad, place it over the drawsheet in the proper area. Not all agencies use drawsheets routinely. The nurse may decide to use one.	
___	___	___	11. Tuck bottom sheet securely under the head of the mattress on one side of the bed, making a corner according to agency policy. A mitered corner is shown in the illustrations. Using a fitted bottom sheet eliminates the need to	

Excellent	Satisfactory	Needs Practice	

Procedure 36-3

Making an Unoccupied Bed (continued)

Goal: To promote a comfortable bed environment when bed is unoccupied.

COMMENTS

			miter corners. Tuck remaining bottom sheet and drawsheet securely under mattress. (At this point, before moving to the other side of the bed, top linens may be placed on the bed, unfolded, and secured, allowing the entire side of the bed to be completed at one time, as shown in the illustrations.)
___	___	___	12. Move to the other side of the bed to secure bottom linens. Secure bottom sheet under the head of the mattress and miter the corner. Pull remainder of the sheet tightly and tuck under mattress. Do the same for the drawsheet.
___	___	___	13. Place top sheet on bed with its center fold in the center of the bed and with the top of the sheet placed so that the hem is even with the head of the mattress. Unfold top sheet in place, as illustrated. Follow same procedure with top blanket or spread, placing upper edge about 6 inches below top of the sheet.
___	___	___	14. Tuck top sheet and blanket under foot of bed on the near side. Miter corners.
___	___	___	15. Fold upper 6 inches of the top sheet down over the spread and make a cuff.
___	___	___	16. Move to other side of bed and follow the same procedure for securing top sheets under the foot of the bed and making a cuff.
___	___	___	17. Place pillows on the bed. Open each pillowcase in the same manner as opening other linens. Gather pillowcase over one hand toward the closed end. Grasp pillow with hand inside the pillowcase. Keeping a firm hold on top of pillow, pull cover onto pillow.
___	___	___	18. Place pillow at the head of the bed with the open end facing toward the window.
___	___	___	19. Fan-fold or pie-fold top linens.
___	___	___	20. Secure signal device on the bed according to agency policy.
___	___	___	21. Adjust bed to the low position.
___	___	___	22. Dispose of soiled linen according to agency policy. Wash your hands.

Procedure Checklists to Accompany Taylor Fundamentals of Nursing: The Art and Science of Nursing Care, 4th Edition

Name _____   Date _____

Unit _____   Position _____

Instructor/Evaluator _____   Position _____

Procedure 36-4

Making an Occupied Bed

Goal: To provide a comfortable bed environment when bed is occupied.

Excellent	Satisfactory	Needs Practice		COMMENTS
▼	▼	▼		
___	___	___	1. Explain procedure to patient. Check patient's chart for limitations on patient's physical activity.	
___	___	___	2. Wash your hands.	
___	___	___	3. Assemble equipment and arrange on bedside chair in the order items will be used.	
___	___	___	4. Close door or curtain.	
___	___	___	5. Adjust patient's bed to the high position. Lower side rail nearest you, leaving opposite side rail up. Place bed in the flat position unless contraindicated.	
___	___	___	6. Check bed linens for patient's personal items and disconnect call bell or any tubes from bed linens.	
___	___	___	7. Place a bath blanket, if available, over patient. Have patient hold onto bath blanket while you reach under it and remove top linens. Leave top sheet in place if a bath blanket is not used. Fold linen that is to be reused over the back of a chair. Discard soiled linen in laundry bag or hamper.	
___	___	___	8. If possible and if another person is available to assist, grasp mattress securely and shift it up to the head of the bed.	
___	___	___	9. Assist patient to turn toward the opposite side of the bed and reposition pillow under patient's head.	
___	___	___	10. Loosen all bottom linens from the head and sides of the bed.	
___	___	___	11. Fan-fold soiled linens as close to patient as possible.	
___	___	___	12. Use clean linen and make the near side of bed following Actions 9, 10, and 11 of Procedure 36-3. Fan-fold clean linen as close to patient as possible.	

Excellent ▼	Satisfactory ▼	Needs Practice ▼	**Procedure 36-4** **Making an Occupied Bed (continued)** **Goal:** To provide a comfortable bed environment when bed is occupied.	COMMENTS
____	____	____	13. Raise side rail. Assist patient to roll over the folded linen in the middle of the bed toward you. Move to other side of bed and lower side rail.	
____	____	____	14. Loosen and remove all bottom linen. Place in a linen bag or hamper. Hold soiled linen away from your uniform.	
____	____	____	15. Ease the clean linen from under the patient. Pull taut and secure bottom sheet under the head of the mattress. Miter corners. Pull side of the sheet taut and tuck under side of the mattress. Repeat this with drawsheet.	
____	____	____	16. Assist patient to return to the center of the bed. Remove pillow and change pillowcases before replacing with open end facing the window.	
____	____	____	17. Apply top linen so that it is centered and top hems are even with the head of the mattress. Have patient hold onto the top linen so bath blanket can be removed.	
____	____	____	18. Secure top linens under foot of mattress and miter corners. Loosen top linens over patient's feet by grasping them in the area of the feet and pulling gently toward the foot of the bed.	
____	____	____	19. Raise side rail. Lower bed height and adjust head of the bed to a comfortable position. Reattach call bell and drainage tubes.	
____	____	____	20. Dispose of soiled linens according to agency policy. Wash your hands.	

Procedure Checklists to Accompany Taylor Fundamentals of Nursing: The Art and Science of Nursing Care, 4ᵗʰ Edition

Name _____ Date _____

Unit _____ Position _____

Instructor/Evaluator _____ Position _____

Excellent ▼	Satisfactory ▼	Needs Practice ▼	*Procedure 36-5* **Assisting Patient with Oral Care** **Goal:** To assist with mechanical cleaning of oral cavity.	COMMENTS
___	___	___	1. Explain procedure to patient.	
___	___	___	2. Wash your hands. Don disposable gloves if assisting with oral care.	
___	___	___	3. Assemble equipment on overbed table within patient's reach.	
___	___	___	4. Provide privacy for patient.	
___	___	___	5. Lower side rail and assist patient to sitting position, if permitted, or turn patient onto the side. Place towel across patient's chest. Raise bed to a comfortable working position.	
___	___	___	6. Encourage patient to brush own teeth or assist if necessary.	
___	___	___	a. Moisten toothbrush and apply toothpaste to bristles.	
___	___	___	b. Place brush at a 45° angle to gum line and brush from gum line to crown of each tooth. Brush outer and inner surfaces. Brush back and forth across biting surface of each tooth.	
___	___	___	c. Brush tongue gently with toothbrush.	
___	___	___	d. Have patient rinse vigorously with water and spit into emesis basin. Repeat until clear. Suction may be used as an alternative for removing fluid and secretions from mouth.	
___	___	___	e. Assist patient to floss teeth, if necessary.	
___	___	___	f. Offer mouthwash if patient prefers.	
___	___	___	7. Assist patient with removal and cleansing of dentures if necessary.	
___	___	___	a. Apply gentle pressure with 4 × 4 gauze to grasp and remove upper denture plate. Place it immediately in denture cup. Lift lower denture using slight rocking motion, remove, and place in denture cup.	

Procedure 36-5

Assisting Patient with Oral Care
(continued)

COMMENTS

Excellent	Satisfactory	Needs Practice		
▼	▼	▼		

___ ___ ___   b. If patient prefers, add denture cleanser with water in a cup and follow preparation directions or brush all areas thoroughly with toothbrush and paste. Place paper towels or washcloth in sink while brushing.

___ ___ ___   c. Rinse thoroughly with water and return dentures to patient.

___ ___ ___   d. Offer mouthwash so patient can rinse mouth before replacing dentures.

___ ___ ___   e. Apply petroleum jelly to lips, if necessary.

___ ___ ___   8. Remove equipment and assist patient to a position of comfort. Record any unusual bleeding or inflammation. Raise side rail and lower bed.

___ ___ ___   9. Remove disposable gloves from inside out and discard appropriately. Wash your hands.

Procedure Checklists to Accompany Taylor Fundamentals of Nursing: The Art and Science of Nursing Care, 4th Edition

Name _____ Date _____

Unit _____ Position _____

Instructor/Evaluator _____ Position _____

Procedure 36-6

Providing Oral Care for the Dependent Patient

Goal: To provide mechanical cleaning of oral cavity for a helpless patient.

Excellent	Satisfactory	Needs Practice		COMMENTS
▼	▼	▼		
___	___	___	1. Explain procedure to patient.	
___	___	___	2. Wash your hands and don disposable gloves.	
___	___	___	3. Assemble equipment on overbed table within reach.	
___	___	___	4. Provide privacy for patient. Adjust bed height to a comfortable position. Lower one side rail and position patient on the side with the head of the bed lowered. Place towel across patient's chest and emesis basin in position under chin.	
___	___	___	5. Open patient's mouth and gently insert a padded tongue blade between back molars, if necessary.	
___	___	___	6. If teeth are present, brush carefully with toothbrush and paste. Remove dentures, if present, and clean before replacing. (See Action 7 of Procedure 36-5.) Use a toothette or gauze-padded tongue blade moistened with normal saline or diluted mouthwash solution to gently cleanse gums, mucous membranes, and tongue.	
___	___	___	7. Use gauze-padded tongue blade dipped in mouthwash solution to rinse oral cavity. If desired, insert rubber tip of irrigating syringe into patient's mouth and rinse gently with a small amount of water. Position patient's head to allow for return of water or use suction apparatus to remove the water from oral cavity.	
___	___	___	8. Apply petroleum jelly to patient's lips.	
___	___	___	9. Remove equipment and return patient to a comfortable position. Raise side rail and lower bed. Record any unusual bleeding or inflammation.	
___	___	___	10. Wash your hands.	

Procedure Checklists to Accompany Taylor Fundamentals of Nursing: The Art and Science of Nursing Care, 4ᵗʰ Edition

Name _____ Date _____

Unit _____ Position _____

Instructor/Evaluator _____ Position _____

Procedure 37-1

Cleaning a Wound and Applying a Dressing

Goal: To promote wound healing and protect wound from injury.

Excellent	Satisfactory	Needs Practice		COMMENTS
▼	▼	▼		
——	——	——	1. Explain procedure to patient.	
——	——	——	2. Gather equipment.	
——	——	——	3. Wash your hands.	
——	——	——	4. Check physician's order for dressing change. Note if drain is present.	
——	——	——	5. Close door or curtain. Use bath blanket as needed when exposing area to be redressed. Position waterproof pad under patient if desired.	
——	——	——	6. Assist patient to comfortable position that provides easy access to wound area.	
——	——	——	7. Place opened, cuffed plastic bag near working area.	
——	——	——	8. Loosen tape on dressing. Use adhesive remover, if necessary. If tape is soiled, don gloves.	
——	——	——	9. Don clean disposable gloves. Remove soiled dressings carefully in a clean to less-clean direction. Do not reach over wound. Check position of drains before removing dressing. If dressing adhers to skin surface, moisten by pouring a small amount of sterile saline onto it. Keep soiled side of dressing away from patient's view.	
——	——	——	10. Assess amount, type, and odor of drainage.	
——	——	——	11. Discard dressings in plastic disposal bag. Pull off glove inside out and drop it in bag.	
——	——	——	12. Using aseptic technique, open sterile dressings, and supplies on work area.	
——	——	——	13. Open sterile cleaning solution and pour over gauze sponges in plastic container or over sponges placed in sterile basin.	

Procedure 37-1

Cleaning a Wound and Applying a Dressing (continued)

Goal: To promote wound healing and protect wound from injury.

Excellent	Satisfactory	Needs Practice		COMMENTS
▼	▼	▼		
——	——	——	14. Don sterile gloves.	
——	——	——	15. Clean wound or surgical incision. Use sterile forceps if desired.	
——	——	——	a. Clean from top to bottom or from center outward.	
——	——	——	b. Use one gauze square for each wipe, discarding each square by dropping into plastic bag. Do not touch bag with forceps.	
——	——	——	c. Clean around drain, if present, moving from center outward in a circular motion. Use one gauze square for each circular motion.	
——	——	——	d. Dry wound using gauze sponge and same motion.	
——	——	——	e. Apply antiseptic ointment, if ordered.	
——	——	——	16. Apply a layer of dry, sterile dressings over wound. Use sterile forceps if desired.	
——	——	——	17. Use sterile scissors to cut sterile 4 × 4 gauze square to place under and around drain if one is present or use precut sterile gauze.	
——	——	——	18. Apply second gauze layer to wound site.	
——	——	——	19. Place surgi-pad or ABD dressing over wound at outermost area.	
——	——	——	20. Remove gloves from inside out and discard them in plastic waste bag. Apply tape or tie existing tapes to secure dressings.	
——	——	——	21. Wash hands. Remove all equipment. Make patient comfortable.	
——	——	——	22. Check dressing and wound site every shift. Record dressing change, wound appearance, and describe any drainage in chart.	

Procedure Checklists to Accompany Taylor Fundamentals of Nursing: The Art and Science of Nursing Care, 4th Edition

Name _____ Date _____

Unit _____ Position _____

Instructor/Evaluator _____ Position _____

Procedure 37-2

Collecting a Wound Culture

Goal: To collect wound drainage for laboratory analysis of microorganisms that cause infection.

Excellent	Satisfactory	Needs Practice		COMMENTS
▼	▼	▼		
___	___	___	1. Explain procedure to patient.	
___	___	___	2. Gather equipment.	
___	___	___	3. Wash your hands.	
___	___	___	4. Don clean disposable gloves. Remove dressings and assess wound and drainage. (See Procedure 37-1, Actions 5–11.)	
___	___	___	5. Using aseptic technique, don sterile gloves and clean wound. (See Procedure 37-1, Action 15.) Remove sterile gloves.	
___	___	___	6. Twist cap to loosen swab in Culturette tube, or open separate swab and remove cap from culture tube, keeping inside uncontaminated.	
___	___	___	7. Don clean glove or new sterile glove, if necessary.	
___	___	___	8. Carefully insert swab into drainage and roll gently. Use another swab if collecting specimen from another site.	
___	___	___	9. Place swab in Culturette tube, being careful not to touch outside of container. Twist cap to secure.	
___	___	___	10. If using Culturette tube, crush ampule of medium at bottom of tube.	
___	___	___	11. Remove gloves from inside out and discard them in plastic waste bag.	
___	___	___	12. Wash your hands.	
___	___	___	13. Apply clean dressing to wound. (See Procedure 37-1, Actions 16-20.)	
___	___	___	14. Wash your hands. Remove all equipment and make patient comfortable.	

Procedure 37-2

Collecting a Wound Culture (continued)

Goal: To collect wound drainage for laboratory analysis of microorganisms that cause infection.

Excellent	Satisfactory	Needs Practice		COMMENTS
▼	▼	▼		
——	——	——	15. Label specimen container appropriately (patient's name, date, time, nature of specimen). Attach laboratory requisition to tube with rubber band or place tube in plastic bag with requisition attached. Send to laboratory within 20 minutes.	
——	——	——	16. Record specimen collection, wound appearance, and description of drainage in chart.	

Procedure Checklists to Accompany Taylor Fundamentals of Nursing: The Art and Science of Nursing Care, 4ᵗʰ Edition

Name _____ Date _____

Unit _____ Position _____

Instructor/Evaluator _____ Position _____

Procedure 37-3

Irrigating a Sterile Wound

Goal: To direct flow of solution into wound
to clean area of pathogens and debris.

Excellent	Satisfactory	Needs Practice		COMMENTS
▼	▼	▼		
—	—	—	1. Explain procedure to patient. Check physician's order for irrigation.	
✓	—	—	2. Gather equipment.	
✓	—	—	3. Wash your hands.	
✓	—	—	4. Close door or curtain. Use bath blanket as needed when exposing wound site.	
—	✓	—	5. Position patient so irrigating solution will flow from upper end of wound toward lower end. Place waterproof pad under patient.	
✓	—	—	6. Warm sterile irrigating solution to body temperature.	
✓	—	—	7. Place opened, cuffed plastic bag near working area. Don gown and goggles if recommended.	
✓	—	—	8. Loosen tape on dressing. Put on clean gloves to remove soiled dressings.	
✓	—	—	9. Assess amount, type, and odor of drainage. Observe wound condition.	
✓	—	—	10. Discard dressings in plastic disposal bag. Remove gloves inside out and drop in bag.	
✓	—	—	11. Using aseptic technique, open sterile dressings and supplies on work area.	
✓	—	—	12. Pour warmed sterile irrigating solution into sterile container. Amount may vary from 200 to 500 mL depending on size of wound.	
✓	—	—	13. Put on sterile gloves. (See Procedure 27-3.)	
✓	—	—	14. Position sterile basin below wound to collect irrigation fluid with nondominant hand.	

Procedure 37-3

Irrigating a Sterile Wound (continued)

Goal: To direct flow of solution into wound
to clean area of pathogens and debris.

Excellent	Satisfactory	Needs Practice		COMMENTS
✓	—	—	15. Use dominant hand to fill syringe with irrigant. Gently direct a stream of solution into wound, keeping tip of syringe 1 inch (2.5 cm) above upper tip of wound. If using a catheter tip on syringe, insert it gently into wound to point of resistance.	
✓	—	—	16. Continue irrigation until solution returns clear. Try to maintain a steady flow of solution.	
✓	—	—	17. Dry area around wound with a sterile gauze sponge.	
✓	—	—	18. Apply layers of sterile dressing.	
✓	—	—	19. Remove gloves and discard them in plastic waste bag. Apply tape to secure dressings.	
✓	—	—	20. Wash hands. Remove all equipment. Make patient comfortable.	
✓	—	—	21. Check dressing and wound site every shift. Record dressing change, wound appearance, and describe any drainage in chart.	

Procedure Checklists to Accompany Taylor Fundamentals of Nursing: The Art and Science of Nursing Care, 4th Edition

Name _____ Date _____

Unit _____ Position _____

Instructor/Evaluator _____ Position _____

Excellent	Satisfactory	Needs Practice	
▼	▼	▼	*Procedure 37-4* **Applying an External Heating Device** **Goal:** To promote wound healing and facilitate comfort through vasodilation and improved blood flow.

				COMMENTS
___	___	___	1. Explain procedure to patient.	
___	___	___	2. Assess skin condition where heat is to be applied.	
___	___	___	3. Assemble necessary equipment. Close door or curtain if privacy is desired.	
___	___	___	4. Wash your hands.	

Hot Water Bag

___	___	___	5. Check water temperature with bath thermometer or test on inner wrist. Rinse bag with water, empty, and then fill.	
___	___	___	6. Fill hot water bag one-half to two-thirds full.	
___	___	___	7. Expel remaining air from bag in one of two ways: Place bag on a flat surface, permit water to come to the opening, then close bag; or hold bag up, twist unfilled portion to remove air, then close bag. Fasten top securely. Check for leaks.	
___	___	___	8. Cover bag with towel or other protector. Apply hot water bottle to prescribed area.	
___	___	___	9. Assess skin condition and patient's response to heat at frequent intervals. Do not exceed prescribed length of time for heat application. Remove hot water bag if excessive swelling, redness, or pain occurs and report to physician.	
___	___	___	10. After removal, record patient's response and dispose of equipment appropriately.	
___	___	___	11. Wash your hands.	

Aquathermia Pad

___	___	___	12. Check that distilled water is at appropriate level. Use key to adjust temperature at 40.6° C (105° F) if it has not already been preset. Plug in unit and warm pad before use.	

Procedure 37-4

Applying an External Heating Device (continued)

Excellent ▼	Satisfactory ▼	Needs Practice ▼	**Goal:** To promote wound healing and facilitate comfort through vasodilation and improved blood flow.	COMMENTS
——	——	——	13. Cover pad with pillowcase or other protector. Apply pad to prescribed area. Do not allow patient to lie on pad if applying to back. Patient should assume prone position and place aquathermia pad on back.	
——	——	——	14. Secure with gauze bandage or tape. Never use safety pins to hold pad in place.	
——	——	——	15. Repeat Actions 9–11.	

Procedure Checklists to Accompany Taylor Fundamentals of Nursing: The Art and Science of Nursing Care, 4th Edition

Name _____ Date _____

Unit _____ Position _____

Instructor/Evaluator _____ Position _____

Procedure 37-5

Applying Warm Sterile Compresses to an Open Wound

Goal: To promote wound healing, improve circulation, and reduce edema.

Excellent	Satisfactory	Needs Practice		COMMENTS
▼	▼	▼		
____	____	____	1. Assess patient for any circulatory impairment at area where compress is to be applied (numbness, tingling, impairment in temperature sensation, or cyanosis).	
____	____	____	2. Check physician's order for warm compresses. Explain procedure to patient.	
____	____	____	3. Gather equipment.	
____	____	____	4. Wash your hands.	
____	____	____	5. Close door or curtain. Use bath blanket as needed when exposing area for application of warm compresses. Position waterproof pad under patient.	
____	____	____	6. Assist patient to comfortable position that provides easy access to area.	
____	____	____	7. Place opened, cuffed plastic bag near working area.	
____	____	____	8. Prepare aquathermia pad or external heating device (optional).	
____	____	____	9. Using sterile technique, open dressings, and warmed solution. Pour solution into sterile container and carefully drop gauze for compresses into sterile solution.	
____	____	____	10. Don clean disposable glove. Remove any dressing carefully and discard in disposable plastic bag. Pull off soiled glove inside out and drop it in bag.	
____	____	____	11. Assess wound healing or presence of infection.	
____	____	____	12. Don sterile gloves.	
____	____	____	13. Retrieve sterile compress from warmed solution and squeeze moisture from it. Apply carefully and gently mold around wound. Be alert for patient's response to heat.	

Procedure 37-5

Applying Warm Sterile Compresses to an Open Wound (continued)

Goal: To promote wound healing, improve circulation, and reduce edema.

Excellent ▼	Satisfactory ▼	Needs Practice ▼		COMMENTS
——	——	——	14. Cover gauze compresses with dry bath towel. Secure in place, if necessary.	
——	——	——	15. Apply aquathermia pad or external heating device over towel (optional).	
——	——	——	16. Monitor skin condition and patient's response to warm compress at frequent intervals.	
——	——	——	17. After 30 minutes (or time ordered by physician), remove warm compress. Carefully observe skin condition around wound and patient's response to application of heat.	
——	——	——	18. Apply sterile dressing to wound. (See Procedure 37-1.)	
——	——	——	19. Dispose of equipment appropriately. Wash hands.	
——	——	——	20. Record patient's response and condition of wound and surrounding skin area.	

Procedure Checklists to Accompany Taylor Fundamentals of Nursing: The Art and Science of Nursing Care, 4th Edition

Name _____ Date _____

Unit _____ Position _____

Instructor/Evaluator _____ Position _____

Excellent	Satisfactory	Needs Practice	
▼	▼	▼	**Procedure 38-1** **Turning a Patient in Bed** **Goal:** To promote comfort and maintain proper body alignment.

Excellent	Satisfactory	Needs Practice		COMMENTS
___	___	___	1. Explain procedure to patient.	
___	___	___	2. Wash your hands.	
___	___	___	3. Raise bed to your waist level. Adjust to flat position or as low as the patient can tolerate. Lower side rail nearest you and raise opposite side.	
___	___	___	4. Position patient closer to the far side of the bed in the supine position.	
___	___	___	5. Place patient's arms across chest and cross patient's far leg over the near one.	
___	___	___	6. Stand opposite the patient's center with your feet spread and one foot ahead of the other. Tighten your gluteal and abdominal muscles and flex your knees.	
___	___	___	7. Position your hands on the patient's far shoulder and hip and roll patient toward you.	
___	___	___	8. Make patient comfortable and position in proper alignment.	
___	___	___	9. Readjust bed height and position and raise side rail if appropriate.	
___	___	___	10. Wash your hands.	

Procedure Checklists to Accompany Taylor Fundamentals of Nursing: The Art and Science of Nursing Care, 4ᵗʰ Edition

Name _____ Date _____

Unit _____ Position _____

Instructor/Evaluator _____ Position _____

Excellent ▼	Satisfactory ▼	Needs Practice ▼	*Procedure 38-2* **Assisting with Passive Range-of-Motion (ROM) Exercises** **Goal:** To move each joint through its range of motion to promote mobility and improve circulation.	COMMENTS
——	——	——	1. Explain procedure to patient.	
——	——	——	2. Wash your hands.	
——	——	——	3. Raise bed to your waist level. Adjust to flat position or as low as patient can tolerate.	
——	——	——	4. Begin ROM exercises at the patient's head and move down one side of the body at a time.	
——	——	——	5. Perform each exercise two to five times, moving each joint in a smooth and rhythmic manner.	
——	——	——	6. Protect joint during ROM exercise.	
——	——	——	7. Progress through ROM exercises for each joint.	
			Head	
——	——	——	• *Flexion*—Move chin down to rest on chest.	
——	——	——	• *Extension*—Return head to normal upright position	
——	——	——	• *Lateral flexion*—Tilt head as far as possible toward each shoulder.	
			Neck	
——	——	——	• *Rotation*—Move head from side to side bringing chin toward shoulder.	
			Shoulder	
——	——	——	• *Flexion*—Start with arm at side and lift arm forward to above head.	
——	——	——	• *Extension*—Return arm to starting position at side of body.	
——	——	——	• *Abduction*—Start with arm at side and move laterally to upright position above head.	

Procedure 38-2

Assisting with Passive Range-of-Motion (ROM) Exercises (continued)

Goal: To move each joint through its range of motion to promote mobility and improve circulation.

Excellent	Satisfactory	Needs Practice		COMMENTS
▼	▼	▼		
——	——	——	• *Adduction*—Lower arm to original position and move across body as far as possible.	
——	——	——	• *Internal and external rotation*—Raise arm at side until upper arm is on line with shoulder. Bend elbow at a 90° angle and move forearm upward and downward.	
			Elbow	
——	——	——	• *Flexion*—Bend elbow and move lower arm and hand upward toward shoulder.	
——	——	——	• *Extension*—Return lower arm and hand to original position while straightening elbow.	
			Forearm	
——	——	——	• *Supination*—Rotate lower arm and hand so palm is up.	
——	——	——	• *Pronation*—Rotate lower arm and hand so palm is down.	
			Wrist	
——	——	——	• *Flexion*—Move hand downward toward inner aspect of forearm.	
——	——	——	• *Extension*—Return hand to neutral position even with forearm.	
——	——	——	• *Hyperextension*—Move dorsal (upper) portion of hand backward as far as possible.	
			Fingers	
——	——	——	• *Flexion*—Bend fingers to make a fist.	
——	——	——	• *Extension*—Straighten fingers.	
——	——	——	• *Abduction*—Spread fingers apart.	
——	——	——	• *Adduction*—Return fingers until they are together.	
——	——	——	• *Opposition of thumb to fingers*—Touch thumb to each finger on hand.	
			Hip	
——	——	——	• *Flexion*—With leg extended, lift upward.	
——	——	——	• *Extension*—Return leg to original position next to other leg.	
——	——	——	• *Abduction*—Lift leg laterally away from body.	

Procedure 38-2

Assisting with Passive Range-of-Motion (ROM) Exercises (continued)

Goal: To move each joint through its range of motion to promote mobility and improve circulation.

Excellent ▼	Satisfactory ▼	Needs Practice ▼		COMMENTS
___	___	___	• *Adduction*—Return leg toward other leg and lift beyond it if possible.	
___	___	___	• *Internal rotation*—Turn foot and leg toward other leg.	
___	___	___	• *External rotation*—Move foot and leg outward away from other leg.	
			Knee	
___	___	___	• *Flexion*—Bend leg bringing heel toward back of leg.	
___	___	___	• *Extension*—Return leg to straight position.	
			Ankle	
___	___	___	• *Dorsiflexion*—Move foot up and back until toes are upright	
___	___	___	• *Plantar flexion*—Move foot with toes pointing downward.	
___	___	___	• *Inversion*—Turn sole of foot toward the middle.	
___	___	___	• *Eversion*—Turn sole of foot outward.	
			Toes	
___	___	___	• *Flexion*—Curl toes downward.	
___	___	___	• *Extension*—Straighten toes out.	
___	___	___	• *Abduction*—Spread toes apart.	
___	___	___	• *Adduction*—Bring toes together.	
___	___	___	8. Return patient to comfortable position.	
___	___	___	9. Readjust bed height and position and raise side rail if it is appropriate.	
___	___	___	10. Wash your hands.	

Procedure Checklists to Accompany Taylor Fundamentals of Nursing: The Art and Science of Nursing Care, 4ᵗʰ Edition

Name _____ Date _____

Unit _____ Position _____

Instructor/Evaluator _____ Position _____

Procedure 38-3

Assisting Patient Up in Bed (Two Nurses)

Goal: To promote comfort, improve circulation, and maintain proper body alignment.

Excellent	Satisfactory	Needs Practice		COMMENTS
▼	▼	▼		
——	——	——	1. Explain procedure to patient.	
——	——	——	2. Wash your hands.	
——	——	——	3. Raise bed to a comfortable position for you. Adjust bed to flat position if patient can tolerate it. With two nurses on opposite sides of bed, lower side rails.	
——	——	——	4. Remove pillow and place it at head of bed.	
——	——	——	5. Place drawsheet on bed under patient's mid-section.	
——	——	——	6. If able to assist, have patient flex knees and place feet flat on bed.	
——	——	——	7. Fold patient's arms across chest and instruct patient to flex neck with chin on chest.	
——	——	——	8. Stand opposite patient's center with your feet spread and turned toward head of bed. Position one foot slightly forward.	
——	——	——	9. Fold or bunch drawsheet close to patient prior to grasping it securely and preparing to move patient.	
——	——	——	10. Shift your weight back and forth from back leg to front leg, and on count of three, move patient upward in bed. If possible, patient can assist the move upward by pushing with his/her legs.	
——	——	——	11. Assist patient to a comfortable position. Reposition pillow. Raise side rail and adjust bed position if necessary.	
——	——	——	12. Wash your hands.	

Procedure Checklists to Accompany Taylor Fundamentals of Nursing: The Art and Science of Nursing Care, 4th Edition

Name _____ Date _____

Unit _____ Position _____

Instructor/Evaluator _____ Position _____

Excellent	Satisfactory	Needs Practice	*Procedure 38-4* # Transferring Patient from Bed to Stretcher **Goal:** To promote safety and prevent patient injury.	COMMENTS
▼	▼	▼		
___	___	___	1. Explain procedure to patient.	
___	___	___	2. Wash your hands.	
___	___	___	3. Move bed and equipment in room to make room for stretcher. Make sure that assistants are available. Close door or curtain.	
___	___	___	4. Raise bed to the same height as the stretcher and adjust head of the bed to the flat position if patient can tolerate it. Lower side rails.	
___	___	___	5. Place drawsheet under patient if one is not already there. Use drawsheet to move patient to the side of the bed where stretcher will be placed.	
___	___	___	6. Position stretcher next to the bed and parallel to it. Lock wheels on stretcher and bed. Remove pillow from bed and place it on stretcher.	
			7. To move patient:	
___	___	___	a. First nurse should kneel on far side of bed away from stretcher. Position knee at the upper torso closer to the patient than the other knee. Grasp drawsheet securely.	
___	___	___	b. Second nurse should reach across stretcher and grasp drawsheet at the patient's head and chest areas.	
___	___	___	c. Third nurse should reach across stretcher and grasp drawsheet at the patient's waist and thigh area. Ask patient to fold arms across chest.	
___	___	___	d. At a signal given by the first nurse, the second and third nurses pull while the first nurse lifts patient from bed to stretcher.	
___	___	___	8. Secure patient on stretcher until side rails are raised. Assist patient to a comfortable position with the covering in place. Leave drawsheet in place for transfer back to bed.	
___	___	___	9. Wash your hands.	

Procedure Checklists to Accompany Taylor Fundamentals of Nursing: The Art and Science of Nursing Care, 4ᵗʰ Edition

Name _____ Date _____

Unit _____ Position _____

Instructor/Evaluator _____ Position _____

Procedure 38-5

Assisting Patient to Transfer from Bed to Chair

Goal: To promote safety, prevent injury, and maintain body alignment.

Excellent	Satisfactory	Needs Practice		COMMENTS
—	—	—	1. Explain procedure to patient. Offer bedpan.	
—	—	—	2. Wash your hands.	
—	—	—	3. Assess patient's ability to assist with transfer. Move equipment as necessary to make room for chair. Close door or curtain.	
—	—	—	4. Place bed in the low position.	
—	—	—	5. Assist patient to put on robe and slippers with nonskid soles.	
—	—	—	6. Position chair at bedside:	
—	—	—	a. *For patient with unimpaired mobility:* Bring chair close to bedside facing foot of bed and, if possible, brace back of chair against bedside table.	
—	—	—	b. *For patient with impaired mobility:* Position chair facing head or foot of bed. When sitting on the side of the bed, patient should be able to steady self by using hand on the unaffected side to grasp arm of chair.	
—	—	—	7. Lock wheels of chair and bed if appropriate. Raise foot pedals on wheelchair to the up position.	
—	—	—	8. Raise head of bed to the highest position.	
—	—	—	9. Assist patient to sit on the side of the bed by supporting patient's head and neck while moving patient's legs off the bed to dangle. Steady patient in that position for a few minutes.	

Procedure 38-5

Assisting Patient to Transfer from Bed to Chair (continued)

Goal: To promote safety, prevent injury, and maintain body alignment.

Excellent	Satisfactory	Needs Practice		COMMENTS
▼	▼	▼		

___	___	___	10. Assist patient to standing position:	
___	___	___	a. *For patient with unimpaired mobility:* Face patient and brace your feet and knees against the patient. Place your hands around patient's waist while patient holds onto you between shoulders and waist. Use your legs to help you raise patient to a standing position.	
___	___	___	b. *For patient with impaired mobility:* Face patient and brace your feet and knees against patient, especially against the affected extremity. Place your hands around patient's waist. Patient may place unaffected arm around your shoulder or use unaffected arm to push up while raising to standing position.	
___	___	___	11. Pivot patient (on unaffected limb if applicable) into a position in front of chair with legs positioned against chair.	
___	___	___	12. Patient may use one arm (unaffected limb, if applicable) to place on the arm of the chair and steady self while slowly lowering to sitting position. Continue to brace patient's knees with your knees and flex your own hips and knees when seating patient.	
___	___	___	13. Adjust patient's position using pillows where necessary. Cover patient and use restraint if necessary. Position call bell so it is available for use.	
___	___	___	14. Wash your hands.	
___	___	___	15. Document patient's tolerance of the procedure and length of time in chair.	

Procedure Checklists to Accompany Taylor Fundamentals of Nursing: The Art and Science of Nursing Care, 4ᵗʰ Edition

Name _____ Date _____

Unit _____ Position _____

Instructor/Evaluator _____ Position _____

Procedure 38-6

Transferring Dependent Patient from Bed to Chair (Two Nurses)

Goal: To promote safety, prevent injury, and maintain body alignment for patient requiring total assistance.

Excellent	Satisfactory	Needs Practice		COMMENTS
▼	▼	▼		
——	——	——	1. Explain procedure to patient.	
——	——	——	2. Wash your hands.	
——	——	——	3. Move equipment as necessary to make room for chair. Close door or curtain. Help patient put on robe and slippers.	
——	——	——	4. Move patient to the nearest side of the bed and cross patient's arms across chest if possible. Lock wheels of the bed.	
——	——	——	5. Position chair next to the bed near the upper end and with back of chair parallel to the head of the bed. (If wheelchair, remove armrest closer to the bed if possible.) Lock wheels, if appropriate.	
——	——	——	6. Adjust bed to a comfortable level for nurses or at the level of the armrest if one is present on chair.	
——	——	——	7. Prepare to lift patient from bed to chair:	
——	——	——	a. First nurse should stand behind the chair. Slip arms under patient's axillae and grasp patient's wrists securely.	
——	——	——	b. Second nurse should face wheelchair and support patient's knees by placing arms under them.	
——	——	——	c. On a predetermined signal, both nurses flex their hips and knees and simultaneously lift patient gently to the chair.	
——	——	——	8. Adjust patient's position using pillows where necessary. Cover patient and use restraint if necessary. Position call bell so it is available for use.	
——	——	——	9. Wash your hands.	
——	——	——	10. Document patient's tolerance of procedure and length of time in chair.	

Procedure Checklists to Accompany Taylor Fundamentals of Nursing: The Art and Science of Nursing Care, 4ᵗʰ Edition

Name _____ Date _____

Unit _____ Position _____

Instructor/Evaluator _____ Position _____

Procedure 40-1

Giving a Back Massage

Excellent	Satisfactory	Needs Practice	**Goal:** To promote comfort and relaxation.	COMMENTS
▼	▼	▼		
____	____	____	1. Explain procedure and offer back massage to patient.	
____	____	____	2. Wash your hands.	
____	____	____	3. Close curtain or door.	
____	____	____	4. Assist patient to the prone position or sidelying position with the back exposed from the shoulders to the sacral area. Use bath blanket to drape patient. Raise bed to the highest position and lower side rail closest to you.	
____	____	____	5. Warm lubricant or lotion in your palm or place container in warm water.	
____	____	____	6. Using light, gliding strokes (effleurage), apply lotion to patient's shoulders, back, and sacral area.	
____	____	____	7. Place your hands beside each other at the base of patient's spine and stroke upward to shoulders and back; downward to buttocks in slow, continuous strokes. Continue for several minutes, applying additional lotion as necessary.	
____	____	____	8. Massage patient's shoulders, entire back, areas over iliac crests and sacrum with circular stroking motion. Keep your hands in contact with patient's skin. Continue for several minutes, applying additional lotion as necessary.	
____	____	____	9. Knead patient's skin by gently alternating grasping and compression motions (petrissage).	
____	____	____	10. Complete massage with additional long stroking movements.	
____	____	____	11. During massage, observe patient's skin for reddened or open areas. Pay particular attention to skin over bony prominences.	
____	____	____	12. Use towel to pat patient dry and to remove excess lotion. Apply powder if patient requests it.	
____	____	____	13. Wash your hands.	
____	____	____	14. Assess patient's response and record your observations on patient's chart.	

Procedure Checklists to Accompany Taylor Fundamentals of Nursing: The Art and Science of Nursing Care, 4ᵗʰ Edition

Name _____ Date _____

Unit _____ Position _____

Instructor/Evaluator _____ Position _____

Procedure 41-1

Inserting Nasogastric Tube

Goal: To pass a tube into the gastrointestinal tract for administration of a formula containing adequate nutrients.

Excellent	Satisfactory	Needs Practice		COMMENTS
▼	▼	▼		
——	——	——	1. Check physician's order for insertion of nasogastric tube.	
——	——	——	2. Explain procedure to patient.	
——	——	——	3. Gather equipment.	
——	——	——	4. If nasogastric tube is rubber, place it in a basin with ice for 5–10 minutes or place a plastic tube in a basin of warm water.	
——	——	——	5. Assess patient's abdomen.	
——	——	——	6. Wash your hands. Don disposable gloves.	
——	——	——	7. Assist patient to high Fowler's position, or 45° if unable to maintain upright position and drape his/her chest with bath towel or disposable pad. Have emesis basin and tissues handy.	
——	——	——	8. Check nares for patency by asking patient to occlude one nostril and breathe normally through the other. Select nostril through which air passes more easily.	
——	——	——	9. Measure distance to insert the tube by placing tip of tube at patient's nostril and extending to tip of earlobe and then to tip of xiphoid process. Mark tube with a piece of tape.	
——	——	——	10. Lubricate tip of tube with water-soluble lubricant. Apply topical analgesic to nostril and oropharynx or ask patient to hold ice chips in his mouth for several minutes (according to physician's preference).	
——	——	——	11. Ask patient to lift his/her head. Insert tube into nostril while directing tube downward and backward. Patient may gag when tube reaches the pharynx.	
——	——	——	12. Instruct patient to keep head in upright or normal eating position. Encourage him/her to swallow even if no fluids are permitted. Advance tube in a downward-and-backward direction when patient swallows. Stop when patient	

Procedure 41-1

Inserting Nasogastric Tube (continued)

Goal: To pass a tube into the gastrointestinal tract for administration of a formula containing adequate nutrients.

Excellent ▼	Satisfactory ▼	Needs Practice ▼		COMMENTS
			breathes. Provide tissues for tearing or watering eyes. If gagging and coughing persist, check placement of tube with a tongue blade and flashlight. Keep advancing tube until tape marking is reached. Do not use force. Rotate tube if it meets resistance.	
——	——	——	13. Discontinue procedure and remove tube if there are signs of distress, such as gasping, coughing, cyanosis, and inability to speak or hum.	
——	——	——	14. Determine that tube is in patient's stomach (these methods are appropriate for large-bore tubes but may be ineffective to check placement of small-bore, pliable tubes):	
——	——	——	a. Attach syringe to end of tube and aspirate a small amount of stomach contents.	
——	——	——	b. Measure pH of aspirated fluid using pH paper or a meter.	
——	——	——	c. Obtain x-ray of placement of tube (as ordered by physician).	
——	——	——	15. Apply tincture of benzoin to tip of nose and allow to dry. Secure tube with tape to patient's nose. Be careful not to pull tube too tightly against nose.	
——	——	——	a. Cut a 4-inch piece of tape and split bottom 2 inches, or use packaged nose tape for NG tubes.	
——	——	——	b. Place unsplit end over bridge of patient's nose.	
——	——	——	c. Wrap split ends under tubing and up and over onto nose.	
——	——	——	16. Attach tube to suction or clamp tube and cap it according to physician's orders.	
——	——	——	17. Secure tube to patient's gown by using a rubber band or tape and a safety pin. If double-lumen tube is used, secure vent above stomach level. Attach at shoulder level.	
——	——	——	18. Assist or provide patient with oral hygiene at regular intervals.	
——	——	——	19. Wash hands. Remove all equipment and make patient comfortable.	
——	——	——	20. Record the insertion procedure, type and size of tube, and measure tube from tip of nose to end of tube. Also document description of gastric contents and patient's response.	

Procedure Checklists to Accompany Taylor Fundamentals of Nursing: The Art and Science of Nursing Care, 4ᵗʰ Edition

Name _____ Date _____

Unit _____ Position _____

Instructor/Evaluator _____ Position _____

Procedure 41-2

Administering Tube Feeding

Goal: To provide enteral nutrition by administering formula at prescribed rate or interval.

Excellent	Satisfactory	Needs Practice		COMMENTS
▼	▼	▼		
____	____	____	1. Explain procedure to patient. Use stethoscope to assess bowel sounds.	
____	____	____	2. Assemble equipment. Check amount, concentration, type, and frequency of tube feeding on patient's chart. Check expiration date of formula.	
____	____	____	3. Wash your hands. Don disposable gloves.	
____	____	____	4. Position patient with head of bed elevated at least 30° or as near normal position for eating as possible.	
____	____	____	5. Unpin tube from patient's gown and check to see that nasogastric tube is properly located in stomach, as described in Procedure 41-1, Action 14.	
____	____	____	6. Aspirate all gastric contents with syringe and measure. Return immediately through tube, saving small amount to measure gastric pH. Flush tube with 30 mL of sterile water for irrigation. Proceed with feeding if amount of residual does not exceed policy of agency or physician's guideline. Disconnect syringe from tubing.	
____	____	____	7. Measure pH of aspirated gastric fluid.	
			For Intermittent Feedings:	
____	____	____	8. When using a feeding bag (open system):	
____	____	____	a. Hang bag on IV pole and adjust to about 12 inches above stomach. Clamp tubing.	
____	____	____	b. Cleanse top of feeding container with alcohol before opening it. Pour formula into feeding bag and allow solution to run through tubing. Close clamp.	
____	____	____	c. Attach feeding set-up to feeding tube, open clamp, and regulate drip according to physician's order or allow feeding to run in over 30 minutes.	

Procedure 41-2

Administering Tube Feeding (continued)

Goal: To provide enteral nutrition by administering formula at prescribed rate or interval.

Excellent	Satisfactory	Needs Practice		COMMENTS
▼	▼	▼		

Excellent	Satisfactory	Needs Practice		
___	___	___	d. Add 30–60 mL (1–2 oz.) of sterile water for irrigation to feeding bag when feeding is almost completed and allow it to run through tube.	
___	___	___	e. Clamp tubing immediately after water has been instilled. Disconnect from tube. Clamp tube and cover end with sterile gauze secured with rubber band or apply cap.	
___	___	___	9. When using prefilled tube feeding set-up (closed system):	
___	___	___	a. Remove screw-on cap and attach administration set-up with drip chamber and tubing. Hang set on IV pole and adjust to about 12 inches above the stomach. Clamp tubing and squeeze drip chamber to fill to 1/3–1/2 of capacity. Release clamp and run formula through tubing. Close clamp.	
___	___	___	b. Follow Actions 8c, 8d, and 8e. Feeding pump may be used with tube feeding set-up to regulate drip.	
			For Continuous Feedings:	
___	___	___	10. When using a feeding pump:	
___	___	___	a. Close flow regulator clamp on tubing and fill feeding bag with prescribed formula. Amount depends on agency policy. Place label on container.	
___	___	___	b. Hang feeding container on IV pole and allow solution to flow through tubing.	
___	___	___	c. Connect to feeding pump following manufacturer's directions. Set rate.	
___	___	___	d. Check residual every 4–8 hours.	
___	___	___	11. Observe patient's response during and after tube feeding.	
___	___	___	12. Have patient remain in upright position for at least 30–60 minutes after feeding.	
___	___	___	13. Wash and clean equipment or replace according to agency policy. Remove gloves and wash your hands.	
___	___	___	14. Record type and amount of feeding and patient's response. Monitor blood glucose, if ordered by physician.	

Procedure Checklists to Accompany Taylor Fundamentals of Nursing: The Art and Science of Nursing Care, 4ᵗʰ Edition

Name _____ Date _____

Unit _____ Position _____

Instructor/Evaluator _____ Position _____

Procedure 41-3

Removing Nasogastric Tube

Goal: To promote comfort and prevent trauma to gastrointestinal tract.

Excellent	Satisfactory	Needs Practice		COMMENTS
▼	▼	▼		
―	―	―	1. Check physician's order for removal of nasogastric tube.	
―	―	―	2. Explain procedure to patient and assist to semi-Fowler's position.	
―	―	―	3. Gather equipment.	
―	―	―	4. Wash your hands. Don clean disposable gloves.	
―	―	―	5. Place towel or disposable pad across patient's chest. Give tissues to patient.	
―	―	―	6. Discontinue suction and separate tube from suction. Unpin tube from patient's gown and carefully remove adhesive tape from patient's nose.	
―	―	―	7. Attach syringe and flush with 10 mL normal saline solution or clear with 30–50 cc of air (optional).	
―	―	―	8. Instruct patient to take a deep breath and hold it.	
―	―	―	9. Clamp tube with fingers by doubling tube on itself. Quickly and carefully remove tube while patient holds breath.	
―	―	―	10. Place tube in disposable plastic bag. Remove gloves and place in bag.	
―	―	―	11. Offer mouth care to patient and facial tissues to blow nose.	
―	―	―	12. Measure nasogastric drainage. Remove all equipment and dispose according to agency policy. Wash your hands.	
―	―	―	13. Record removal of tube, patient's response, and measure of drainage. Continue to monitor patient for 2–4 hours after tube removal for gastric distention, nausea, or vomiting.	

Procedure Checklists to Accompany Taylor Fundamentals of Nursing: The Art and Science of Nursing Care, 4ᵗʰ Edition

Name _____ Date _____

Unit _____ Position _____

Instructor/Evaluator _____ Position _____

Procedure 41-4

Irrigating Nasogastric Tube Connected to Suction

Goal: To maintain patency of gastrointestinal tube.

Excellent	Satisfactory	Needs Practice		COMMENTS
▼	▼	▼		
___	___	___	1. Check physician's order for irrigation. Explain procedure to patient.	
___	___	___	2. Gather necessary equipment. Check expiration dates on irrigating saline solution and irrigation set.	
___	___	___	3. Wash your hands.	
___	___	___	4. Assist patient to semi-Fowler's position, unless this is contraindicated.	
___	___	___	5. Check placement of nasogastric tube. (Refer to Procedure 41-1, Action 14.)	
___	___	___	6. Pour irrigating solution into container. Draw up 30 mL of saline solution (or amount ordered by physician) into syringe.	
___	___	___	7. Clamp suction tubing near connection site. Disconnect tube from suction apparatus and lay on disposable pad or towel, or hold both tubes upright in nondominant hand.	
___	___	___	8. Place tip of syringe in tube. If Salem sump or double-lumen tube is used, make sure that syringe tip is placed in drainage port and not in air vent. Hold syringe upright and gently insert the irrigant (or allow solution to flow in by gravity, if agency or physician indicates). Do not force solution into tube.	
___	___	___	9. If unable to irrigate tube, reposition patient and attempt irrigation again. Check with physician if repeated attempts to irrigate tube fail.	
___	___	___	10. Withdraw or aspirate fluid into syringe. If no return, inject 20 cc of air and aspirate again.	
___	___	___	11. Reconnect tube to suction. Observe movement of solution or drainage.	

Procedure 41-4

Irrigating Nasogastric Tube Connected to Suction (continued)

Excellent ▼	Satisfactory ▼	Needs Practice ▼	**Goal:** To maintain patency of gastrointestinal tube.	COMMENTS
____	____	____	12. Measure and record amount and description of irrigant and returned solution.	
____	____	____	13. Rinse equipment if it will be reused.	
____	____	____	14. Wash your hands.	
____	____	____	15. Record irrigation procedure, description of drainage, and patient's response.	

Procedure Checklists to Accompany Taylor Fundamentals of Nursing: The Art and Science of Nursing Care, 4th Edition

Name _____ Date _____

Unit _____ Position _____

Instructor/Evaluator _____ Position _____

Procedure 41-5

Monitoring Blood Glucose Level

Excellent	Satisfactory	Needs Practice	**Goal:** To measure serum blood glucose levels.	COMMENTS
▼	▼	▼		
___	___	___	1. Check physician's order for monitoring schedule.	
___	___	___	2. Gather equipment.	
___	___	___	3. Explain procedure to patient.	
___	___	___	4. Wash hands. Don disposable gloves.	
___	___	___	5. Prepare lancet.	
___	___	___	6. Remove test strip from vial and recap container immediately. Turn monitor on and check that code number on strip matches code number on monitor screen.	
___	___	___	7. Massage side of finger for adult (or heel for child) toward puncture site.	
___	___	___	8. Have patient wash hands with soap and warm water or cleanse area with alcohol. Dry thoroughly.	
___	___	___	9. With finger in dependent position, hold lancet perpendicular to skin and prick side of fingerpad with lancet.	
___	___	___	10. Wipe away first drop of blood with cotton ball if recommended by manufacturer of monitor.	
___	___	___	11. Lightly squeeze or milk puncture site until a hanging drop of blood has formed. (Check instructions for monitor.)	
___	___	___	12. Gently touch drop of blood to pad on test strip without smearing it.	
___	___	___	13. Insert strip into meter according to directions for that specific device. Some devices require that the drop of blood be applied to a test strip already inserted in monitor.	
___	___	___	14. Press timer if directed by manufacturer.	
___	___	___	15. Apply pressure to puncture site.	
___	___	___	16. Read blood glucose results and document appropriately at bedside. Inform patient of test result.	

Excellent	Satisfactory	Needs Practice	
▼	▼	▼	

Procedure 41-5

Monitoring Blood Glucose Level (continued)

Goal: To measure serum blood glucose levels.

COMMENTS

Excellent	Satisfactory	Needs Practice	
——	——	——	17. Turn off meter. Dispose of supplies appropriately. Place lancet in sharps container.
——	——	——	18. Remove gloves and wash hands.
——	——	——	19. Record blood glucose on chart or medication record.

Procedure Checklists to Accompany Taylor Fundamentals of Nursing: The Art and Science of Nursing Care, 4th Edition

Name _____ Date _____

Unit _____ Position _____

Instructor/Evaluator _____ Position _____

Procedure 42-1

Offering and Removing Bedpan or Urinal

Goal: To provide privacy while assisting a bedridden patient to void or defecate.

Excellent	Satisfactory	Needs Practice		COMMENTS
▼	▼	▼		
____	____	____	1. Bring bedpan or urinal and equipment to bedside. Don disposable gloves.	
____	____	____	2. Warm bedpan, if it is made of metal, by rinsing with warm water.	
____	____	____	3. Place adjustable bed in the high position.	
____	____	____	4. Place bedpan or urinal on chair next to bed or on foot of bed. Fold top linen back just enough to allow placement of bedpan or urinal.	
____	____	____	5. If patient needs assistance to move onto bedpan, have him/her bend knees and rest some of his/her weight on heels. Lift patient by placing one hand under lower back and slip bedpan into place with the other hand.	
____	____	____	6. If patient is helpless, two people may be required to lift him/her onto bedpan. Or patient may be placed on his/her side, bedpan placed against buttocks, and patient rolled back onto bedpan.	
____	____	____	7. When bedpan is in its proper place, patient's buttocks rest on the rounded shelf of bedpan. For male patients, urinal is properly placed between slightly spread legs with penis positioned in it and with urinal resting on bed.	
____	____	____	8. If permitted, raise head of the bed as near to the sitting position as tolerated.	
____	____	____	9. Place call device and toilet tissue within easy reach. Leave patient if it is safe to do so. Use side rails appropriately.	

Procedure 42-1

Offering and Removing Bedpan or Urinal (continued)

Goal: To provide privacy while assisting a bedridden patient to void or defecate.

Excellent	Satisfactory	Needs Practice		COMMENTS
▼	▼	▼		
——	——	——	10. Remove bedpan in the same manner in which it was offered, being careful to hold it steady. If necessary to assist patient, don disposable gloves, wrap tissue around the hand several times, and wipe patient clean, using one stroke from the pubic area toward the anal area. Discard tissue and use more until patient is clean. Place patient on his/her side and spread buttocks to clean anal area. Cover bedpan.	
——	——	——	11. Do not place toilet tissue in bedpan if a specimen is required or if measurement of elimination is required. Have receptacle handy for discarding tissue.	
——	——	——	12. Offer patient supplies to wash and dry his/her hands, assisting as necessary.	
——	——	——	13. Empty and clean bedpan and urinal. Wash your hands. Record according to agency procedure.	

Procedure Checklists to Accompany Taylor Fundamentals of Nursing: The Art and Science of Nursing Care, 4ᵗʰ Edition

Name _____ Date _____

Unit _____ Position _____

Instructor/Evaluator _____ Position _____

Procedure 42-2

Catheterizing the Female Urinary Bladder (Straight and Indwelling)

Goal: To safely introduce catheter into bladder to promote urine drainage.

Excellent	Satisfactory	Needs Practice		COMMENTS
▼	▼	▼		
____	____	____	1. Assemble equipment. Wash your hands. Explain procedure and purpose to patient.	
____	____	____	2. Provide good light. Artificial light is recommended (use of flashlight requires an assistant to hold and position it).	
____	____	____	3. Provide privacy by closing curtains or door.	
____	____	____	4. Assist patient to the dorsal recumbent position with knees flexed and feet about 2 feet apart. Drape patient. Or, if preferable, place patient in the side-lying position. Slide waterproof drape under patient.	
____	____	____	5. Clean genital and perineal areas with warm soap and water. Rinse and dry. Wash your hands again.	
____	____	____	6. Prepare urine drainage setup if indwelling catheter is to be inserted and separate urine collection system is used. Secure to bed frame according to manufacturer's directions.	
____	____	____	7. Open sterile catheterization tray on overbed table using sterile technique.	
____	____	____	8. Put on sterile gloves. Grasp upper corners of drape and unfold without touching unsterile areas. Fold back cuff over gloved hands. Ask patient to lift her buttocks. Slide sterile drape under her with gloves protected by cuff.	
____	____	____	9. Fenestrated sterile drape may be placed over perineal area exposing the labia.	
____	____	____	10. Place sterile tray on drape between patient's thighs.	

Procedure 42-2

Catheterizing the Female Urinary Bladder (Straight and Indwelling) (continued)

Goal: To safely introduce catheter into bladder to promote urine drainage.

Excellent	Satisfactory	Needs Practice		COMMENTS
▼	▼	▼		
___	___	___	11. Open all supplies:	
___	___	___	a. *If catheter is to be indwelling:* Test catheter balloon. Remove protective cap on tip of syringe and attach syringe prefilled with sterile water to injection port. Inject appropriate amount of fluid. If balloon inflates properly, withdraw fluid and leave syringe attached to port.	
___	___	___	b. Pour antiseptic solution over cotton balls or gauze. Open specimen container if specimen is to be obtained.	
___	___	___	c. Lubricate 1–2 inches of catheter tip.	
___	___	___	12. With thumb and one finger of your nondominant hand, spread labia and identify meatus. Be prepared to maintain separation of labia with one hand until urine is flowing well and continuously.	
___	___	___	13. Using cotton balls held with forceps, clean both labial folds then directly over meatus. Move cotton ball from above the meatus down toward the rectum. Discard each cotton ball after one downward stroke.	
___	___	___	14. With uncontaminated gloved hand, place drainage end of the catheter in receptacle. For *insertion of an indwelling catheter* that is preattached to sterile tubing and drainage container (closed drainage system), position catheter and setup within easy reach on the sterile field.	
___	___	___	15. Insert catheter tip into the meatus 5–7.5 cm (2–3 inches) or until urine flows. Do not use force to push catheter through the urethra into the bladder. Ask patient to breathe deeply. Rotate catheter gently if slight resistance is met as catheter reaches the external sphincter. *For an indwelling catheter:* Once urine drains, advance catheter another 2.5–5.0 cm (1–2 inches).	
___	___	___	16. Hold catheter securely with the nondominant hand while bladder empties. Collect specimen if required. Continue drainage according to agency policy.	
___	___	___	17. Remove catheter smoothly and slowly if a straight catheterization was ordered.	

Procedure 42-2

Catheterizing the Female Urinary Bladder (Straight and Indwelling) (continued)

Goal: To safely introduce catheter into bladder to promote urine drainage.

Excellent	Satisfactory	Needs Practice		COMMENTS
▼	▼	▼		
___	___	___	18. *If the catheter is to be indwelling:*	
___	___	___	a. Inflate balloon according to manufacturer's recommendations.	
___	___	___	b. Tug gently on catheter after balloon is inflated to feel resistance.	
___	___	___	c. Attach catheter to drainage system if necessary.	
___	___	___	d. Secure to upper thigh with a Velcro leg strap or tape. Leave some slack in catheter to allow for leg movement.	
___	___	___	e. Check that drainage tubing is not kinked and that movement of side rails does not interfere with catheter or drainage bag.	
___	___	___	19. Remove equipment and make patient comfortable in bed. Clean and dry perineal area, if necessary. Care for equipment according to agency policy. Send urine specimen to laboratory promptly or refrigerate it.	
___	___	___	20. Wash your hands.	
___	___	___	21. Record time of catheterization, amount of urine removed, description of urine, patient's reaction to procedure, and your name.	

Procedure Checklists to Accompany Taylor Fundamentals of Nursing: The Art and Science of Nursing Care, 4th Edition

Name _____ Date _____

Unit _____ Position _____

Instructor/Evaluator _____ Position _____

Procedure 42-3

Catheterizing the Male Urinary Bladder (Straight and Indwelling)

Goal: To safely introduce catheter into bladder to promote urine drainage.

Excellent	Satisfactory	Needs Practice		COMMENTS
▼	▼	▼		
___	___	___	1. Assemble equipment and follow Actions 1–3 for female catheterization in Procedure 42-2.	
___	___	___	2. Position patient on his back with thighs slightly apart. Drape patient so that only area around penis is exposed.	
___	___	___	3. Follow Actions 5–7 for female catheterization in Procedure 42-2.	
___	___	___	4. Put on sterile gloves. Open sterile drape and place on patient's thighs. Place fenestrated drape with opening over penis.	
___	___	___	5. Place catheter set on or next to patient's legs on the sterile drape.	
___	___	___	6. Open all supplies:	
___	___	___	a. *If catheter is to be indwelling:* Test catheter balloon. Remove protective cap on tip of syringe and attach syringe prefilled with sterile water to the injection port. Inject appropriate amount of fluid. If balloon inflates properly, withdraw fluid, and leave syringe attached to port.	
___	___	___	b. Pour antiseptic solution over cotton balls or gauze. Open specimen container if specimen is to be obtained.	
___	___	___	c. Remove cap from syringe prefilled with lubricant.	
___	___	___	7. Lift penis with your nondominant hand, which is then considered contaminated. Retract foreskin in the uncircumcised male patient. Clean area at meatus with cotton ball held with forceps. Use circular motion, moving from meatus toward base of penis for three cleansings.	

Procedure 42-3

Catheterizing the Male Urinary Bladder (Straight and Indwelling) (continued)

Excellent ▼ **Satisfactory** ▼ **Needs Practice** ▼

Goal: To safely introduce catheter into bladder to promote urine drainage.

COMMENTS

___ ___ ___   8. Hold penis with slight upward tension and perpendicular to patient's body. Gently insert tip of syringe with lubricant into urethra and instill 10 mL of lubricant.

___ ___ ___   9. Ask patient to bear down as if voiding. With your dominant hand, place drainage end of catheter in the receptacle. *For insertion of indwelling catheter* that is preattached to sterile tubing and drainage container (closed drainage system), position catheter and setup within easy reach on the sterile field.

___ ___ ___   10. Insert tip into meatus. Advance catheter 15–20 cm (6–8 inches) or until urine flows. Do not use force to introduce catheter. If catheter resists entry, ask patient to breathe deeply and rotate catheter slightly. *For indwelling catheter,* once urine drains, advance catheter to the bifurcation of the catheter. Once balloon is inflated, catheter may be gently pulled back into place. Lower penis.

___ ___ ___   11. Follow Actions 16 through 21 for female catheterization in Procedure 42-2 except that catheter may be secured to upper thigh or lower abdomen with penis directed toward patient's chest. Slack should be left in catheter to prevent tension.

Procedure Checklists to Accompany Taylor Fundamentals of Nursing: The Art and Science of Nursing Care, 4ᵗʰ Edition

Name _____ Date _____

Unit _____ Position _____

Instructor/Evaluator _____ Position _____

Procedure 42-4

Irrigating Catheter Using the Closed System

Goal: To restore or maintain patency of an indwelling catheter through intermittent flushing of the tube.

Excellent	Satisfactory	Needs Practice		COMMENTS
▼	▼	▼		
——	——	——	1. Assemble equipment. Wash your hands. Explain procedure and purpose to patient.	
——	——	——	2. Provide privacy by closing curtains or door and draping patient with bath blanket.	
——	——	——	3. Assist patient to a comfortable position and expose aspiration port on catheter setup. Place waterproof drape under catheter and aspiration port.	
——	——	——	4. Open sterile supplies. Pour sterile solution into sterile basin. Aspirate irrigant (30–50 mL) into the sterile syringe and attach capped sterile needle. Don gloves.	
——	——	——	5. Disinfect aspiration port with alcohol swabs or gauze square with antiseptic solution.	
——	——	——	6. Clamp or fold catheter tubing distal to aspiration port.	
——	——	——	7. Remove cap and insert needle into port. Gently instill solution into catheter.	
——	——	——	8. Remove needle from port. Unclamp tubing and allow irrigant and urine to drain. Repeat procedure as necessary.	
——	——	——	9. Assess patient's response to procedure and quality and amount of drainage. Document on patient's chart.	
——	——	——	10. Record amount of irrigant used on intake-output record. Subtract this from urine output when totaled.	
——	——	——	11. Remove equipment and discard uncapped needle and syringe in appropriate receptacle. Remove gloves and wash your hands. Make patient comfortable.	

Procedure Checklists to Accompany Taylor Fundamentals of Nursing: The Art and Science of Nursing Care, 4ᵗʰ Edition

Name _____ Date _____

Unit _____ Position _____

Instructor/Evaluator _____ Position _____

Procedure 42-5

Giving Continuous Bladder Irrigation

Goal: To restore or maintain patency of indwelling catheter through continuous flushing of tube.

Excellent	Satisfactory	Needs Practice		COMMENTS
▼	▼	▼		
___	___	___	1. Explain procedure and purpose to patient.	
___	___	___	2. Assemble equipment.	
___	___	___	3. Wash your hands.	
___	___	___	4. Provide privacy by closing curtains or door and draping patient with bath blanket.	
___	___	___	5. Prepare sterile irrigation bag for use as directed by manufacturer. Secure clamp and attach sterile tubing with drip chamber to container. Hang bag on IV pole 2.5–3 feet above level of patient's bladder. Release clamp and remove protective cover on end of tubing without contaminating it. Allow solution to flush tubing and remove air. Reclamp.	
___	___	___	6. Using sterile technique, attach irrigation tubing to the irrigation port of the 3-way Foley catheter. If a closed system is used, tubing may already be connected to irrigation port on catheter.	
___	___	___	7. Release clamp on irrigation tubing and regulate flow according to physician's order.	
___	___	___	8. As irrigation is completed, clamp tubing. Do not allow drip chamber to empty. Disconnect empty bag and attach full irrigation bag. Continue as ordered by physician.	
___	___	___	9. Assess patient's response to procedure and quality and amount of drainage. Document on patient's chart.	
___	___	___	10. Record amount of irrigant used on intake-output record. Don gloves and empty drainage collection bag as each new container is hung. Record.	
___	___	___	11. Wash your hands.	

Procedure Checklists to Accompany Taylor Fundamentals of Nursing: The Art and Science of Nursing Care, 4ᵗʰ Edition

Name _____ Date _____

Unit _____ Position _____

Instructor/Evaluator _____ Position _____

Procedure 42-6

Applying a Condom Catheter

Goal: To safely apply an external device to penis to collect urine.

Excellent ▼	Satisfactory ▼	Needs Practice ▼		COMMENTS
___	___	___	1. Explain procedure to patient. Ask if patient is aware of any allergy to latex.	
___	___	___	2. Assemble equipment. Prepare urinary drainage setup or reusable leg bag for attachment to condom sheath.	
			3. Wash your hands.	
___	___	___	4. Assist patient to the supine position. Close curtain or door. Use bath blanket and sheet to expose only patient's genital area.	
___	___	___	5. Don disposable gloves. Wash genital area with soap and water, rinse, and dry thoroughly.	
___	___	___	6. Roll condom sheath outward onto itself. Grasp penis firmly with your nondominant hand. Apply condom sheath by rolling it onto penis with your dominant hand. Leave a 2.5–5 cm (1–2 inch) space between tip of penis and end of condom sheath.	
___	___	___	7. Apply elastic or Velcro strap in a snug but not tight manner. Do not allow elastic or Velcro to come in contact with skin.	
___	___	___	8. Connect condom sheath to the drainage setup. Avoid kinking or twisting drainage tubing.	
___	___	___	9. Remove equipment. Place patient in a comfortable, safe position. Wash your hands.	
___	___	___	10. Assess patient's response and record observations on patient's record.	

Procedure Checklists to Accompany Taylor Fundamentals of Nursing: The Art and Science of Nursing Care, 4ᵗʰ Edition

Name _____ Date _____

Unit _____ Position _____

Instructor/Evaluator _____ Position _____

Excellent ▼	Satisfactory ▼	Needs Practice ▼	*Procedure 42-7* **Changing Stoma Appliance on an Ileal Conduit** **Goal:** To facilitate urine collection and stoma assessment of a surgically-created urinary diversion.	COMMENTS
——	——	——	1. Explain procedure and encourage patient to observe or participate if possible. Provide for privacy.	
——	——	——	2. Assemble equipment.	
——	——	——	3. Wash your hands and don disposable gloves.	
——	——	——	4. Have patient sit or stand, if able, to assist with procedure or assume supine position in bed.	
——	——	——	5. Empty pouch being worn into graduated container (before removing if it is reusable and not attached to straight drainage).	
——	——	——	6. Gently remove pouch faceplate from skin.	
——	——	——	7. Discard pouch appropriately, if disposable, or wash reusable pouch in lukewarm soap and water and allow to air dry.	
——	——	——	8. Clean skin around stoma with soap and water or commercial cleaner using washcloth or cotton balls. Make sure you remove all old adhesive from skin.	
——	——	——	9. Gently pat dry. Make sure skin around stoma is thoroughly dry. Assess stoma and condition of surrounding skin.	
——	——	——	10. Place a gauze square or two over stoma opening.	
——	——	——	11. Apply skin protectant to a 5-cm (2-inch) radius around stoma and allow it to dry completely, which takes about 30 seconds.	
——	——	——	12. If necessary, enlarge size of faceplate opening to fit stoma.	
——	——	——	13. Apply adhesive to faceplate or remove protective covering from disposable faceplate. Carefully position appliance and press in place, moving from the center outward. Remove gauze squares from stoma before applying pouch.	

Procedure 42-7

Changing Stoma Appliance
on an Ileal Conduit (continued)

Goal: To facilitate urine collection and stoma assessment of a surgically-created urinary diversion.

Excellent ▼	Satisfactory ▼	Needs Practice ▼		COMMENTS
——	——	——	14. Secure optional belt to appliance and around patient.	
——	——	——	15. Remove or discard equipment and assess patient's response to procedure. Wash your hands and remove gloves.	
——	——	——	16. Record appearance of stoma and surrounding skin as well as patient's reaction to procedure.	

Procedure Checklists to Accompany Taylor Fundamentals of Nursing: The Art and Science of Nursing Care, 4th Edition

Name _____ Date _____

Unit _____ Position _____

Instructor/Evaluator _____ Position _____

Procedure 43-1

Administering a Cleansing Enema

Goal: To introduce solution into large intestine to promote expulsion of feces.

Excellent	Satisfactory	Needs Practice		COMMENTS
▼	▼	▼		
___	___	___	1. Assemble necessary equipment. Warm solution in amount ordered and check temperature with a bath thermometer, if available. If tap water is used, adjust temperature as it flows from the tap.	
___	___	___	2. Explain procedure to patient and plan where he/she will defecate. Have bedpan, commode, or nearby bathroom ready for his/her use.	
___	___	___	3. Wash your hands.	
___	___	___	4. Add enema solution to container. Release clamp and allow fluid to progress through tube before reclamping.	
___	___	___	5. Position waterproof pad under patient.	
___	___	___	6. Provide privacy. Position and drape patient on the left side (Sims position) with anus exposed or on back, as dictated by patient comfort and condition.	
___	___	___	7. Put on disposable gloves.	
___	___	___	8. Elevate solution so it is 45 cm (18 inches) above level of patient's anus. Plan to administer solution slowly over a period of 5–10 minutes. Container may be hung on IV pole or held in nurse's hands at the proper height.	
___	___	___	9. Generously lubricate the last 5–7 cm (2–3 inches) of rectal tube. Disposable enema set may have a prelubricated rectal tube.	
___	___	___	10. Lift buttock to expose anus. Slowly and gently insert rectal tube 7–10 cm (3–4 inches). Direct it at an angle pointing toward umbilicus.	
___	___	___	11. If tube meets resistance while inserting it, permit a small amount of solution to enter, withdraw tube slightly, then continue to insert it. Do not force tube entry. Ask patient to take several deep breaths.	

Excellent ▼	Satisfactory ▼	Needs Practice ▼	

Procedure 43-1

Administering a Cleansing Enema (continued)

Goal: To introduce solution into large intestine
to promote expulsion of feces.

COMMENTS

Excellent	Satisfactory	Needs Practice		COMMENTS
___	___	___	12. Introduce solution slowly over a period of 5–10 minutes. Hold tubing all the time solution is being instilled. Commercial preparations may be administered by compressing container with hands according to package directions.	
___	___	___	13. Clamp tubing or lower container if patient has the desire to defecate or cramping occurs. Patient also may be instructed to take small, fast breaths or to pant.	
___	___	___	14. After solution has been given, clamp tubing and remove tube. Have paper towel ready to receive tube as it is withdrawn. Have patient retain solution until the urge to defecate becomes strong, usually in about 5–15 minutes.	
___	___	___	15. Remove disposable gloves from inside out and discard.	
___	___	___	16. When patient has a strong urge to defecate, place him/her in a sitting position on bedpan or assist to commode or bathroom.	
___	___	___	17. Record character of the stool and patient's response to the enema. Remind patient not to flush commode before nurse inspects results of enema.	
___	___	___	18. Assist patient, if necessary, with cleaning of anal area. Offer washcloth, soap, and water to wash his/her hands.	
___	___	___	19. Leave patient clean and comfortable. Care for equipment properly.	
___	___	___	20. Wash your hands.	

Procedure Checklists to Accompany Taylor Fundamentals of Nursing: The Art and Science of Nursing Care, 4th Edition

Name _____   Date _____

Unit _____   Position _____

Instructor/Evaluator _____   Position _____

Procedure 43-2

Changing or Emptying an Ostomy Appliance

Goal: To protect skin surrounding the ostomy site, collect fecal discharge, and control odor.

Columns: Excellent ▼ | Satisfactory ▼ | Needs Practice ▼   COMMENTS

1. Assemble necessary equipment.

2. Explain procedure to patient.

3. Wash your hands and don disposable gloves.

4. Provide for patient's privacy. Assist to a comfortable sitting or lying position in bed or a standing or sitting position in bathroom.

To Change Pouch:

5. Empty partially filled appliance into bedpan if pouch is drainable.

6. Slowly remove appliance, beginning at the top, while keeping abdominal skin taut. If there is any resistance, use warm water or adhesive solvent to facilitate removal. Discard disposable pouch in plastic bag.

7. Use toilet tissue to remove any excess stool from stoma. Cover stoma with a gauze pad. Gently wash and pat dry peristomal skin. Mild soap or a cleansing agent may be used according to agency policy.

8. Assess appearance of peristomal skin and stoma. A moist, reddish-pink stoma is considered normal.

9. Apply skin barrier and appliance together (wafer or disc style):

   a. Select size for stoma opening by using measurement guide.

   b. Trace same size circle on the back and center of skin barrier.

   c. Use scissors to cut an opening 1/4–1/8 inch larger than stoma.

Procedure 43-2

Changing or Emptying
an Ostomy Appliance (continued)

Goal: To protect skin surrounding the ostomy site,
collect fecal discharge, and control odor.

COMMENTS

Excellent	Satisfactory	Needs Practice	
___	___	___	d. Remove backing to expose sticky side.
___	___	___	e. Remove gauze pad covering stoma.
___	___	___	f. Ease barrier and pouch over stoma and gently press onto skin while smoothing out creases or wrinkles. Hold pouch in place for 5 minutes.
___	___	___	10. Close pouch if it is drainable by folding end upward and using clamp or clip. (See manufacturer's directions.)

To Empty Pouch:

___	___	___	11. Plan to drain pouch when it is one-third to one-half full. Remove clamp and fold end of pouch upward like a cuff.
___	___	___	12. Empty contents into bedpan or into toilet. Rinse pouch with tepid water or water mixed with a drop of mouthwash administered via squeeze bottle.
___	___	___	13. Wipe lower 2 inches of pouch with toilet tissue.
___	___	___	14. Uncuff edge of pouch and apply clip or clamp.
___	___	___	15. Dispose of used equipment according to agency policy. Remove gloves and wash hands.
___	___	___	16. Document appearance of stoma, condition of peristomal skin, characteristics of drainage (amount, color, consistency, unusual odor), and patient's reaction to procedure.

Procedure Checklists to Accompany Taylor Fundamentals of Nursing: The Art and Science of Nursing Care, 4th Edition

Name _____ Date _____

Unit _____ Position _____

Instructor/Evaluator _____ Position _____

Procedure 44-1

Using Pulse Oximeter

Goal: To measure oxygen saturation of blood.

Excellent	Satisfactory	Needs Practice		COMMENTS
▼	▼	▼		
____	____	____	1. Explain procedure to patient.	
____	____	____	2. Wash your hands.	
____	____	____	3. Select adequate site for application of sensor:	
____	____	____	a. Use patient's index, middle, or ring finger.	
____	____	____	b. Check proximal pulse and capillary refill at pulse closest to site.	
____	____	____	c. If circulation at site is inadequate, earlobe or bridge of nose may be considered.	
____	____	____	d. Use toe only if lower extremity circulation is not compromised.	
____	____	____	4. Use proper equipment:	
____	____	____	a. If one finger is too large for the probe, use a smaller one.	
____	____	____	b. Use probes appropriate for patient's age and size. A pediatric probe may be used for a small adult.	
____	____	____	c. Check if patient is allergic to adhesive. A nonadhesive finger clip or reflectance sensor is available.	
____	____	____	5. Prepare monitoring site:	
____	____	____	a. Cleanse selected area and allow to dry.	
____	____	____	b. Remove nail polish and artificial nails after checking manufacturer's instructions.	
____	____	____	6. Apply probe securely to skin. Make sure light-emitting sensor and light-receiving sensor are aligned opposite each other (not necessary to check if placed on forehead or bridge of nose).	
____	____	____	7. Connect sensor probe to pulse oximeter and check operation of equipment (presence of audible beep and fluctuation of bar of light or waveform on face of oximeter).	

Excellent ▼	Satisfactory ▼	Needs Practice ▼	*Procedure 44-1* # Using Pulse Oximeter (continued) **Goal:** To measure oxygen saturation of blood.	COMMENTS
___	___	___	8. Set alarms on pulse oximeter. Check manufacturer's alarm limits for high and low pulse rate settings.	
___	___	___	9. Check oxygen saturation at regular intervals as ordered by physician and necessitated by alarms. Monitor patient's hemoglobin level.	
___	___	___	10. Remove sensor on a regular basis and check for skin irritation or signs of pressure (every 2 hrs.; every 4 hrs. for adhesive finger or toe sensor).	
___	___	___	11. Evaluate any malfunctions or problems with equipment.	
___	___	___	a. For absent or weak signal, check patient's vital signs and condition. If satisfactory, check connections and circulation to the site.	
___	___	___	b. For inaccurate reading, check prescribed medications and history of circulatory disorders. Try device on a healthy person to see if problem is equipment-related or patient-related.	
___	___	___	c. If bright light (sunlight or fluorescent light) is suspected of causing equipment malfunction, cover probe with a dry washcloth.	
___	___	___	12. Document and report SaO2 appropriately.	

Procedure Checklists to Accompany Taylor Fundamentals of Nursing: The Art and Science of Nursing Care, 4th Edition

Name _____ Date _____

Unit _____ Position _____

Instructor/Evaluator _____ Position _____

Excellent ▼	Satisfactory ▼	Needs Practice ▼	*Procedure 44-2* # Administering Oxygen by Nasal Cannula **Goal:** To provide oxygen delivery via nasal cannula.	COMMENTS
___	___	___	1. Explain procedure to patient and review safety precautions necessary when oxygen is in use. Place No Smoking signs in appropriate areas.	
___	___	___	2. Wash your hands.	
___	___	___	3. Connect nasal cannula to oxygen setup with humidification, if one is in use. Adjust flow rate as ordered by physician. Check that oxygen is flowing out of prongs.	
___	___	___	4. Place prongs in patient's nostrils. Adjust according to type of equipment:	
___	___	___	a. Over and behind each ear with adjuster comfortably under chin; or	
___	___	___	b. Around patient's head.	
___	___	___	5. Use gauze pads at ear beneath tubing as necessary.	
___	___	___	6. Encourage patient to breathe through nose with mouth closed.	
___	___	___	7. Wash your hands.	
___	___	___	8. Assess and chart patient's response to therapy.	
___	___	___	9. Remove and clean cannula and assess nares at least every 8 hours or according to agency recommendations. Check nares for evidence of irritation or bleeding.	

Name _____ Date _____

Unit _____ Position _____

Instructor/Evaluator _____ Position _____

Excellent	Satisfactory	Needs Practice		
▼	▼	▼	***Procedure 44-3*** # Administering Oxygen by Mask **Goal:** To provide oxygen delivery via a mask apparatus.	**COMMENTS**
___	___	___	1. Explain procedure to patient and review safety precautions necessary when oxygen is in use. Place No Smoking signs in appropriate areas.	
___	___	___	2. Wash your hands.	
___	___	___	3. Attach face mask to oxygen setup with humidification. Start flow of oxygen at specified rate. For a mask with a reservoir, allow oxygen to fill bag before placing mask over patient's nose and mouth.	
___	___	___	4. Position face mask over patient's nose and mouth. Adjust it with elastic strap so mask fits snugly but comfortably on face.	
___	___	___	5. Use gauze pads to reduce irritation on patient's ears and scalp.	
___	___	___	6. Wash your hands.	
___	___	___	7. Remove mask and dry skin every 2–3 hours if oxygen is running continuously. Do not powder around mask.	
___	___	___	8. Assess and chart patient's response to therapy.	

Procedure Checklists to Accompany Taylor Fundamentals of Nursing: The Art and Science of Nursing Care, 4ᵗʰ Edition

Name _____ Date _____

Unit _____ Position _____

Instructor/Evaluator _____ Position _____

Excellent	Satisfactory	Needs Practice	*Procedure 44-4* **Suctioning Nasopharyngeal and Oropharyngeal Areas**	COMMENTS
▼	▼	▼	**Goal:** To remove secretions from oropharyngeal and nasalpharyngeal airways.	
___	___	___	1. Determine need for suctioning. Administer pain medication before suctioning to postoperative patient.	
___	___	___	2. Explain procedure to patient.	
___	___	___	3. Assemble equipment.	
___	___	___	4. Wash your hands.	
___	___	___	5. Adjust bed to comfortable working position. Lower side rail closer to you. Place patient in a semi-Fowler's position if he/she is conscious. An unconscious patient should be placed in the lateral position facing you.	
___	___	___	6. Place towel or waterproof pad across patient's chest.	
___	___	___	7. Turn suction to appropriate pressure:	
___	___	___	a. Wall unit: Adult: 100–120 mmHg Child: 95–110 mmHg Infant: 50–95 mmHg	
___	___	___	b. Portable unit Adult: 10–15 mmHg Child: 5–10 mmHg Infant: 2–5 mmHg	
___	___	___	8. Open sterile suction package. Set up sterile container, touching only the outside surface, and pour sterile water into it.	
___	___	___	9. Don sterile gloves. Dominant hand that will handle catheter must remain sterile while nondominant hand is considered clean rather than sterile.	

Procedure 44-4

Suctioning Nasopharyngeal and Oropharyngeal Areas (continued)

Goal: To remove secretions from oropharyngeal and nasalpharyngeal airways.

Excellent	Satisfactory	Needs Practice		COMMENTS
▼	▼	▼		
——	——	——	10. With sterile gloved hand, pick up sterile catheter and connect to suction tubing held with unsterile hand.	
——	——	——	11. Moisten catheter by dipping it into container of sterile saline. Occlude Y-tube to check suction.	
——	——	——	12. Estimate distance from earlobe to nostril, and place thumb and forefinger of gloved hand at that point on catheter.	
——	——	——	13. Gently insert catheter with suction off by leaving vent on the Y-connector open. Slip catheter gently along the floor of an unobstructed nostril toward trachea to suction the nasopharynx. Or insert catheter along side of mouth toward trachea to suction oropharynx. Never apply suction as catheter is introduced.	
——	——	——	14. Apply suction by occluding suctioning port with your thumb. Gently rotate catheter as it is being withdrawn. Do not allow suctioning to continue for more than 10–15 seconds at a time.	
——	——	——	15. Flush catheter with saline and repeat suctioning as needed and according to patient's toleration of procedure.	
——	——	——	16. Allow at least a 20- to 30-second interval if additional suctioning is needed. Nares should be alternated when repeated suctioning is required. Do not force catheter through nares. Encourage patient to cough and breathe deeply between suctionings.	
——	——	——	17. When suctioning is completed, remove gloves inside out and dispose of gloves, catheter, and container with solution in proper receptacle. Wash your hands.	
——	——	——	18. Use auscultation to listen to chest and breath sounds to assess effectiveness of suctioning.	
——	——	——	19. Record time of suctioning and nature and amount of secretions. Also note character of patient's respirations before and after suctioning.	
——	——	——	20. Offer oral hygiene after suctionings.	

Procedure Checklists to Accompany Taylor Fundamentals of Nursing: The Art and Science of Nursing Care, 4ᵗʰ Edition

Name _____ Date _____

Unit _____ Position _____

Instructor/Evaluator _____ Position _____

Excellent	Satisfactory	Needs Practice	
▼	▼	▼	**Procedure 44-5** **Suctioning the Tracheostomy** **Goal:** To remove secretions from an artificial airway and promote oxygen exchange.

				COMMENTS
___	___	___	1. Explain procedure to patient and reassure him/her that you will interrupt procedure if patient indicates respiratory difficulty. Administer pain medication to postoperative patient before suctioning.	
___	___	___	2. Gather equipment and provide privacy for patient.	
___	___	___	3. Wash your hands.	
___	___	___	4. Assist patient to a semi-Fowler's or Fowler's position if conscious. An unconscious patient should be placed in the lateral position facing you.	
___	___	___	5. Turn suction to appropriate pressure:	

___	___	___	a. Wall unit:
			    Adult: 100–120 mmHg
			    Child: 95–110 mmHg
			    Infant: 50 mmHg	

___	___	___	b. Portable unit:
			    Adult: 10–15 mmHg
			    Child: 5–10 mmHg
			    Infant: 2–5 mmHg	

___	___	___	6. Place clean towel, if being used, across patient's chest. Don goggles, mask, and gown, if necessary.	
___	___	___	7. Open sterile kit or set up equipment and prepare to suction:	
___	___	___	a. Place sterile drape, if available, across patient's chest.	
___	___	___	b. Open sterile container and place on bedside table or overbed table without contaminating inner surface. Pour sterile saline into it.	

Excellent

Satisfactory

Needs Practice

▼   ▼   ▼

Procedure 44-5

Suctioning the Tracheostomy (continued)

Goal: To remove secretions from an artificial airway
and promote oxygen exchange.

COMMENTS

___ ___ ___		c. Hyperoxygenate patient using manual resuscitation bag or sigh mechanism on mechanical ventilator.	
___ ___ ___		d. Don sterile gloves or one sterile glove on dominant hand and clean glove on nondominant hand.	
___ ___ ___		e. Connect sterile suction catheter to suction tubing held with unsterile gloved hand.	
___ ___ ___		8. Moisten catheter by dipping it into container of sterile saline, unless it is one of the newer silicone catheters that does not require lubrication.	
___ ___ ___		9. Remove oxygen delivery setup with unsterile gloved hand if it is still in place.	
___ ___ ___		10. Using sterile gloved hand, gently and quickly insert catheter into the trachea. Advance about 10–12.5 cm (4–5 inches) or until patient coughs. *Do not occlude Y-port when inserting catheter.*	
___ ___ ___		11. Apply intermittent suction by occluding Y-port with thumb of unsterile gloved hand. Gently rotate catheter with thumb and index finger of sterile gloved hand as catheter is being withdrawn. Do not allow suctioning to continue for more than 10 seconds. Hyperventilate 3–5 times between suctionings or encourage patient to cough and deep breathe between suctionings.	
___ ___ ___		12. Flush catheter with saline and repeat suctioning as needed and according to patient's tolerance of procedure. Allow patient to rest at least 1 minute between suctionings, and replace oxygen delivery setup if necessary. Limit suctioning events to three times.	
___ ___ ___		13. When procedure is completed, turn off suction and disconnect catheter from suction tubing. Remove gloves inside out and dispose of gloves, catheter, and container with solution in proper receptacle. Wash hands.	
___ ___ ___		14. Adjust patient's position. Auscultate chest to evaluate breath sounds.	
___ ___ ___		15. Record time of suctioning and nature and amount of secretions. Also note character of patient's respirations before and after suctioning.	
___ ___ ___		16. Offer oral hygiene.	

Procedure Checklists to Accompany Taylor Fundamentals of Nursing: The Art and Science of Nursing Care, 4ᵗʰ Edition

Name _____   Date _____

Unit _____   Position _____

Instructor/Evaluator _____   Position _____

Excellent	Satisfactory	Needs Practice	

Procedure 44-6

Providing Tracheostomy Care

Goal: To clean artificial airway and prevent accumulation of secretions that interfere with oxygenation.

COMMENTS

Excellent	Satisfactory	Needs Practice	
___	___	___	1. Explain procedure to patient.
___	___	___	2. If tracheostomy tube has just been suctioned, remove soiled dressing from around tube and discard with gloves on removal.
___	___	___	3. Wash your hands and open necessary supplies.
			Cleaning Nondisposable Inner Cannula
___	___	___	4. Prepare supplies prior to cleaning inner cannula:
___	___	___	a. Open tracheostomy care kit and separate basins, touching only the edges. If kit is not available, open two sterile basins.
___	___	___	b. Fill one basin 1/2-inch (1.25 cm) deep with hydrogen peroxide.
___	___	___	c. Fill other basin 1/2-inch (1.25 cm) deep with saline.
___	___	___	d. Open sterile brush or pipe cleaners if they are not already in cleaning kit. Open additional sterile gauze pad.
___	___	___	5. Don disposable gloves.
___	___	___	6. Remove oxygen source if one is present. Rotate lock on inner cannula in a counter-clockwise motion to release it.
___	___	___	7. Gently remove inner cannula and carefully drop it in basin with hydrogen peroxide. Remove gloves and discard.
___	___	___	8. Clean inner cannula:
___	___	___	a. Don sterile gloves.
___	___	___	b. Remove inner cannula from soaking solution. Moisten brush or pipe cleaners in saline and insert into tube, using back-and-forth motion.

Procedure 44-6

Providing Tracheostomy Care (continued)

Goal: To clean artificial airway and prevent accumulation of secretions that interfere with oxygenation.

Excellent	Satisfactory	Needs Practice		COMMENTS
—	—	—	c. Agitate cannula in saline solution. Remove and tap against inner surface of basin.	
—	—	—	d. Place on sterile gauze pad.	
—	—	—	9. Suction outer cannula using sterile technique.	
—	—	—	10. Replace inner cannula into outer cannula. Turn lock clockwise and make sure that inner cannula is secure. Reapply oxygen source if needed.	

Replacing Disposable Inner Cannula

Excellent	Satisfactory	Needs Practice		
—	—	—	11. Release lock. Gently remove inner cannula and place in disposable bag. Discard gloves and don sterile ones to insert new cannula. Replace with appropriately sized new cannula. Engage lock on inner cannula.	

Applying Clean Dressing and Tape

Excellent	Satisfactory	Needs Practice		
—	—	—	12. Dip cotton-tipped applicator in saline and clean stoma under faceplate. Use each applicator only once, moving from stoma site outward.	
—	—	—	13. Apply hydrogen peroxide to area around stoma, faceplate, and outer cannula if secretions prove difficult to remove. Rinse area with saline.	
—	—	—	14. Pat skin gently with dry 4 × 4 gauze.	
—	—	—	15. Slide commercially prepared tracheostomy dressing or pre-folded non-cotton-filled 4 × 4 dressing under faceplate.	
—	—	—	16. Change tracheostomy tape:	
—	—	—	a. Leave soiled tape in place until new one is applied.	
—	—	—	b. Cut piece of tape that is twice the neck circumference plus 4 inches (10 cm). Trim ends on the diagonal.	
—	—	—	c. Insert one end of tape through faceplate opening alongside old tape. Pull through until both ends are even.	
—	—	—	d. Slide both tapes under patient's neck and insert one end through remaining opening on other side of faceplate. Pull snugly and tie ends in double square knot. Check that patient can flex neck comfortably.	
—	—	—	e. Carefully remove old tape. Reapply oxygen source if necessary.	
—	—	—	17. Remove gloves and discard. Wash hands. Assess patient's respirations. Document assessments and completion of procedure.	

Procedure Checklists to Accompany Taylor Fundamentals of Nursing: The Art and Science of Nursing Care, 4ᵗʰ Edition

Name _____ Date _____

Unit _____ Position _____

Instructor/Evaluator _____ Position _____

Excellent	Satisfactory	Needs Practice		COMMENTS
▼	▼	▼	**Procedure 45-1** **Starting Intravenous Infusion** **Goal:** To provide a safe route for administration of intravenous therapy.	
___	___	___	1. Gather all equipment and bring to bedside. Check IV solution and medication additives against physician's order.	
___	___	___	2. Explain procedure to patient.	
___	___	___	3. Wash your hands.	
___	___	___	4. Prepare IV solution and tubing:	
___	___	___	a. Maintain aseptic technique when opening sterile packages and IV solution.	
___	___	___	b. Clamp tubing, uncap spike, and insert into entry site on bag as manufacturer directs.	
___	___	___	c. Squeeze drip chamber and allow it to fill at least half way.	
___	___	___	d. Remove cap at end of tubing, release clamp and allow fluid to move through tubing. Allow fluid to flow until all air bubbles have disappeared. Close clamp and recap end of tubing, maintaining sterility of setup.	
___	___	___	e. If electronic device is used, follow manufacturer's instructions for inserting tubing and setting infusion rate.	
			f. Apply label if medication was added to container. (Pharmacy may have added medication and applied label.)	
___	___	___	g. Place time-tape on container.	
___	___	___	5. Place patient in a low Fowler's position in bed. Place protective towel or pad under patient's arm.	
___	___	___	6. Select appropriate site and palpate accessible veins.	
___	___	___	7. If site is hairy and agency policy permits, clip a 2-inch area around intended entry site.	

Excellent ▼	Satisfactory ▼	Needs Practice ▼	*Procedure 45-1* **Starting Intravenous Infusion (continued)**	COMMENTS
			Goal: To provide a safe route for administration of intravenous therapy.	
―	―	―	8. Apply tourniquet 5–6 inches above venipuncture site to obstruct venous blood flow and distend vein. Direct tourniquet ends away from entry site. Check to be sure radial pulse is still present.	
―	―	―	9. Ask patient to open and close his/her fist. Observe and palpate for a suitable vein. Try the following techniques if vein cannot be felt:	
―	―	―	a. Release tourniquet and have patient lower his/her arm below level of heart to fill veins. Reapply tourniquet and gently tap over intended vein to help distend it.	
―	―	―	b. Remove tourniquet and place warm, moist compresses over intended vein for 10–15 minutes.	
―	―	―	10. Don clean gloves.	
―	―	―	11. Cleanse entry site with an antiseptic solution (alcohol swab) followed by antimicrobial solution (povidone iodine) according to agency policy. Use circular motion to move from the center outward for several inches.	
―	―	―	12. Use nondominant hand, placed about 1–2 inches below entry site, to hold skin taut against vein. Avoid touching prepared site.	
―	―	―	13. Enter skin gently with catheter held by the hub in the dominant hand, bevel side up, at a 10–30° angle. Catheter may be inserted from either directly over vein or from side of vein. While following the course of the vein, advance needle or catheter into vein. A sensation of "give" can be felt when needle enters vein.	
―	―	―	14. When blood returns through lumen of needle or flashback chamber of catheter, advance either device 1/8 to 1/4 inch farther into vein. Catheter needs to be advanced until hub is at venipuncture site but exact technique depends on type of device used.	
―	―	―	15. Release tourniquet. Quickly remove protective cap from IV tubing and attach tubing to catheter or needle. Stabilize catheter or needle with nondominant hand.	
―	―	―	16. Start solution flow promptly by releasing clamp on tubing. Examine tissue around entry site for signs of infiltration.	
―	―	―	17. Secure catheter with narrow, non-allergenic tape (1/2 inch) placed sticky side up under hub and crossed over top of hub.	

Procedure 45-1

Starting Intravenous Infusion (continued)

Goal: To provide a safe route for administration of intravenous therapy.

Excellent	Satisfactory	Needs Practice		COMMENTS
▼	▼	▼		
——	——	——	18. Place sterile dressing over venipuncture site. Agency policy may direct nurse to use gauze dressing or transparent dressing. Apply tape to dressing if necessary. Loop tubing near entry site and anchor to dressing.	
——	——	——	19. Mark date, time, site, and type and size of catheter used for infusion on the tape. Anchor tubing.	
——	——	——	20. Anchor arm to an armboard for support, if necessary, or apply site protector or tube-shaped mesh netting over insertion site.	
——	——	——	21. Adjust rate of solution flow according to amount prescribed or follow manufacturer's directions for adjusting flow rate on infusion pump.	
——	——	——	22. Remove all equipment and dispose in proper manner. Remove gloves and wash hands.	
——	——	——	23. Document procedure and patient's response. Chart time, site, device used, and solution.	
——	——	——	24. Return to check flow rate and observe for infiltration 30 minutes after starting infusion.	

Procedure Checklists to Accompany Taylor Fundamentals of Nursing: The Art and Science of Nursing Care, 4th Edition

Name _____ Date _____

Unit _____ Position _____

Instructor/Evaluator _____ Position _____

Procedure 45-2

Changing IV Solution and Tubing

Goal: To safely maintain IV therapy using aseptic technique.

Excellent	Satisfactory	Needs Practice		COMMENTS
▼	▼	▼		
——	——	——	1. Gather all equipment and bring to bedside. Check IV solution and medication additives against physician's order.	
——	——	——	2. Explain procedure to patient.	
——	——	——	3. Wash your hands.	
			To Change IV Solution:	
——	——	——	4. Carefully remove protective cover from new solution container and expose entry site.	
——	——	——	5. Close clamp on tubing.	
——	——	——	6. Lift container off IV pole and invert it. Quickly remove spike from old IV container being careful not to contaminate it.	
——	——	——	7. Steady new container and insert spike. Hang on IV pole.	
——	——	——	8. Reopen clamp on tubing and adjust flow.	
——	——	——	9. Label container according to agency policy. Record on intake-output record and document on chart according to agency policy. Discard used equipment in proper manner. Wash your hands.	
			To Change IV Tubing and Solution:	
——	——	——	10. Follow Actions 1 to 4.	
——	——	——	11. Open administration set and close clamp on new tubing. Remove protective covering from infusion spike. Using sterile technique, insert into new container.	
——	——	——	12. Hang IV container on pole and squeeze drip chamber to fill at least halfway.	
——	——	——	13. Remove cap at end of tubing, release clamp, and allow fluid to move through tubing until all air bubbles have disappeared. Close clamp and recap end of tubing maintaining sterility of setup.	

Procedure 45-2

Changing IV Solution and Tubing (continued)

Goal: To safely maintain IV therapy using aseptic technique.

Excellent	Satisfactory	Needs Practice		COMMENTS
▼	▼	▼		
——	——	——	14. Loosen tape at IV insertion site. Don clean gloves. Carefully remove dressing and tape.	
——	——	——	15. Place sterile gauze square under needle hub.	
——	——	——	16. Place new IV tubing close to patient's IV site and slightly loosen protective cap.	
——	——	——	17. Clamp old IV tubing. Steady needle hub with nondominant hand until change is completed. Remove tubing with dominant hand using a twisting motion. A short closed tubing set with an injection port and closure clamp between needle or angiocath hub and tubing also may be used.	
——	——	——	18. Set old tubing aside. Maintaining sterility, carefully remove cap and insert sterile end of tubing into needle hub. Twist to secure it. Remove soiled gloves.	
——	——	——	19. Open clamp.	
——	——	——	20. Reapply sterile dressing to site according to agency protocol. (See Procedure 45-4.)	
——	——	——	21. Regulate IV flow according to physician's order.	
——	——	——	22. Attach to IV tubing tape or label that states date, time, and your initials. Label container and record procedure, according to agency policy. Discard used equipment in proper manner and wash hands.	
——	——	——	23. Record patient's response to IV infusion.	

Procedure Checklists to Accompany Taylor Fundamentals of Nursing: The Art and Science of Nursing Care, 4ᵗʰ Edition

Name _____ Date _____

Unit _____ Position _____

Instructor/Evaluator _____ Position _____

Excellent ▼	Satisfactory ▼	Needs Practice ▼		COMMENTS
			Procedure 45-3 # Monitoring IV Site and Infusion **Goal:** To provide for safe delivery of prescribed IV fluids.	
——	——	——	1. Monitor IV infusion several times a shift. More frequent checks may be necessary if medication is infused.	
——	——	——	a. Check physician's order for IV solution.	
——	——	——	b. Check drip chamber and time drops if IV is not regulated by an infusion control device.	
——	——	——	c. Check tubing for anything that might interfere with flow. Be sure that clamp is in open position. Observe dressing for leakage of IV solution.	
——	——	——	d. Observe settings, alarm, and indicator lights on infusion control device, if one is being used.	
——	——	——	2. Inspect site for swelling, pain, coolness or pallor at site of injection, which may indicate infiltration of IV. It may become necessary to remove IV and restart at another site.	
——	——	——	3. Inspect IV site for redness, swelling, heat and pain, which may indicate phlebitis is present. Notify physician if you suspect phlebitis may have occurred. It may become necessary to discontinue IV and restart at another site.	
——	——	——	4. Check for local or systemic manifestations that indicate an infection is present at IV site. The IV will be discontinued and the physician notified. Be careful not to disconnect IV tubing when putting on patient's hospital gown.	
——	——	——	5. Be alert for additional complications of IV therapy.	
——	——	——	a. Circulatory overload can result in signs of cardiac failure and pulmonary edema. Monitor I-O during IV therapy.	
——	——	——	b. Bleeding at the site is most likely to occur when IV is discontinued.	

Procedure 45-3

Monitoring IV Site and Infusion (continued)

Excellent	Satisfactory	Needs Practice	
▼	▼	▼	**Goal:** To provide for safe delivery of prescribed IV fluids.

COMMENTS

Excellent	Satisfactory	Needs Practice		
___	___	___	6. If possible, instruct patient to call for assistance if any discomfort is noted at IV site, solution container is nearly empty, or flow has changed in any way.	
___	___	___	7. Document IV infusion, any complications of therapy, and patient's reaction to therapy.	

Procedure Checklists to Accompany Taylor Fundamentals of Nursing: The Art and Science of Nursing Care, 4ᵗʰ Edition

Name _____ Date _____

Unit _____ Position _____

Instructor/Evaluator _____ Position _____

Excellent ▼	Satisfactory ▼	Needs Practice ▼	Procedure 45-4 **Changing an IV Dressing** **Goal:** To control contamination of IV site and prevent introduction of microorganisms into blood stream.	COMMENTS
			Peripheral	
——	——	——	1. Assess patient's need for dressing change.	
——	——	——	2. Gather equipment and bring to bedside. Place towel or disposable pad under extremity.	
——	——	——	3. Explain procedure to patient.	
——	——	——	4. Wash your hands. Don clean gloves.	
——	——	——	5. Carefully remove old dressing but leave tape that anchors IV needle or catheter in place. Discard in proper manner.	
——	——	——	6. Assess IV site for presence of inflammation or infiltration. If noted, discontinue and relocate IV.	
——	——	——	7. Loosen tape and gently remove, being careful to steady catheter or needle hub with one hand. Use adhesive remover if necessary.	
——	——	——	8. Cleanse entry site with an alcohol swab using a circular motion moving from the center outward. Allow to dry. Follow with povidone-iodine swab using the same process.	
——	——	——	9. Reapply tape strip to needle or catheter at entry site.	
——	——	——	10. Apply sterile gauze or transparent polyurethane dressing over entry site. Remove gloves and dispose properly.	
——	——	——	11. Secure IV tubing with additional tape if necessary. Label dressing with date, time of change, and initials. Check that IV flow is accurate and system is patent.	
			Central Venous Access Device	
——	——	——	12. Follow Actions 1–5.	
——	——	——	13. Remove gloves and wash hands thoroughly. If agency requires, nurse and patient should put on a mask. Open dressing kit using sterile technique.	

Procedure 45-4

Changing an IV Dressing (continued)

Excellent ▼	Satisfactory ▼	Needs Practice ▼	**Goal:** To control contamination of IV site and prevent introduction of microorganisms into blood stream.	COMMENTS
___	___	___	14. Put on sterile gloves.	
___	___	___	15. Using alcohol swabs, move in a circular fashion from the insertion site outward (1 1/2–2 inch area). Allow to dry.	
___	___	___	16. Follow alcohol cleansing with povidone-iodine swabs using the same technique. Allow to dry.	
___	___	___	17. Reapply sterile dressing or securement device according to agency policy. Secure tubing or lumens to prevent tugging on insertion site.	
___	___	___	18. Note date, time of dressing change, size of catheter, and initials on tape or dressing.	
___	___	___	19. Discard equipment properly and wash hands.	
___	___	___	20. Record patient's response to dressing change and observation of site.	

Procedure Checklists to Accompany Taylor Fundamentals of Nursing: The Art and Science of Nursing Care, 4ᵗʰ Edition

Name _____ Date _____

Unit _____ Position _____

Instructor/Evaluator _____ Position _____

Procedure 45-5

Capping Primary Line for Intermittent Use

Goal: To provide for intermittent venous access for delivery of prescribed medications.

Excellent	Satisfactory	Needs Practice		COMMENTS
▼	▼	▼		
——	——	——	1. Gather equipment and verify physician's order. Fill lock end extension tubing with normal saline or heparin flush. Recap syringe for use in Action 10.	
——	——	——	2. Explain procedure to patient.	
——	——	——	3. Wash your hands.	
——	——	——	4. Assess IV site.	
——	——	——	5. Clamp off primary line.	
——	——	——	6. Don clean gloves.	
——	——	——	7. Place gauze 4 × 4 sponge underneath IV connection hub between IV catheter and tubing.	
——	——	——	8. Stabilize hub of IV catheter with nondominant hand. Use dominant hand to quickly twist and disconnect IV tubing from catheter, discard it and prefilled lock device or needless cap to hub without contaminating tips of catheter and lock. Extension tubing may be attached.	
——	——	——	9. Cleanse cap with alcohol wipe.	
——	——	——	10. Insert syringe with blunt cannula or standard syringe into heparin lock port and gently flush catheter with saline or heparin flush as per agency policy. Remove syringe carefully.	
——	——	——	11. Tape lock or cap securely in place.	
——	——	——	12. Chart on IV administration record or medication Kardex per institutional policy.	

Procedure Checklists to Accompany Taylor Fundamentals of Nursing: The Art and Science of Nursing Care, 4th Edition

Name _____ Date _____

Unit _____ Position _____

Instructor/Evaluator _____ Position _____

Excellent	Satisfactory	Needs Practice	
▼	▼	▼	**_Procedure 45-6_** # **Administering a Blood Transfusion** **Goal:** To safely infuse blood or blood products into the venous circulation.

COMMENTS

Excellent	Satisfactory	Needs Practice	
____	____	____	1. Determine if patient knows reason for transfusion. Ask if patient has had a transfusion or transfusion reaction in the past.
____	____	____	2. Explain procedure to patient. Make sure there is a signed consent for transfusion, if required by agency. Advise patient to report any chills, itching, rash, or unusual symptoms.
____	____	____	3. Wash your hands and put on clean gloves.
____	____	____	4. Hang container of 0.9% normal saline with blood administration set to initiate IV infusion and follow procedures for administration of blood.
____	____	____	5. Start intravenous with #18 or #19 catheter, if not already present. (See Procedure 45-1.) Keep IV open by starting flow of normal saline.
____	____	____	6. Obtain blood product from blood bank according to agency policy.
____	____	____	7. Complete identification and checks as required by agency:
____	____	____	a. Identification number
____	____	____	b. Blood group and type
____	____	____	c. Expiration date
____	____	____	d. Patient's name
____	____	____	e. Inspect blood for clots.
____	____	____	8. Take baseline set of vital signs prior to beginning transfusion.

Procedure 45-6

Administering a Blood Transfusion (continued)

Goal: To safely infuse blood or blood products into the venous circulation.

Excellent	Satisfactory	Needs Practice		COMMENTS
―	―	―	e. Inspect blood for clots.	
―	―	―	8. Take baseline set of vital signs prior to beginning transfusion.	
			9. Start infusion of blood product:	
			a. Prime in-line filter with blood.	
―	―	―	b. Start administration slowly (no more than 25–50 mL for the first 15 minutes). Stay with patient for first 5–15 minutes of transfusion.	
―	―	―	c. Check vital signs at least every 15 minutes for the first half hour after start of transfusion and then every half-hour or hour after transfusion, depending on agency policy.	
―	―	―	d. Observe patient for flushing, dyspnea, itching, hives, or rash.	
―	―	―	e. Use a blood-warming device, if indicated, especially with rapid transfusions through a CVP catheter.	
―	―	―	10. Maintain prescribed flow rate as ordered or as deemed appropriate by the patient's overall condition, keeping in mind outer limits for safe administration. Assess frequently for transfusion reaction. Stop blood transfusion and allow saline to flow if you suspect a reaction. Notify physician and blood bank.	
			11. When transfusion is complete, infuse 0.9% normal saline.	
			12. Record administration of blood and patient's reaction as ordered by agency. Return blood transfusion bag to blood bank according to agency policy.